Paediatric and Adolescent Gynaecology for the MRCOG and Beyond

WITHDRAWN FROM LIBRARY

Published titles in the MRCOG and Beyond series

Antenatal Disorders for the MRCOG and Beyond *by Andrew Thomson and Ian Greer*

Fetal Medicine for the MRCOG and Beyond *by Alan Cameron, Lena Macara, Janet Brennand and Peter Milton*

Gynaecological and Obstetric Pathology for the MRCOG *by Harold Fox and C. Hilary Buckley, with a chapter on Cervical Cytology by Dulcie V Coleman*

Gynaecological Oncology for the MRCOG and Beyond *edited by David Luesley and Nigel Acheson*

Gynaecological Urology for the MRCOG and Beyond *by Simon Jackson, Meghana Pandit and Alexandra Blackwell*

Haemorrhage and Thrombosis for the MRCOG and Beyond *edited by Anne Harper*

Intrapartum Care for the MRCOG and beyond *by Thomas F. Baskett and Sabaratnam Arulkumaran, with a chapter on Neonatal Resuscitation by John McIntyre and a chapter on Perinatal Loss by Carolyn Basak*

Management of Infertility for the MRCOG and Beyond, second edition, *edited by Siladitya Bhattacharya and Mark Hamilton*

Medical Genetics for the MRCOG and Beyond *by Michael Connor*

Menopause for the MRCOG and Beyond, second edition *by Margaret Rees*

Menstrual Problems for the MRCOG *by Mary Ann Lumsden, Jane Norman and Hilary Critchley*

Neonatology for the MRCOG *by Peter Dear and Simon Newell*

Reproductive Endocrinology for the MRCOG and Beyond, second edition, *edited by Adam Balen*

The MRCOG: A Guide to the Examination, third edition, *edited by William L Ledger*

Forthcoming titles in the series

Early Pregnancy Issues

Molecular Medicine

Paediatric and Adolescent Gynaecology for the MRCOG and Beyond

Second Edition

Anne Garden FRCOG, ILTM
Head of Medicine, Lancaster University;
Honorary Consultant Gynaecologist,
University Hospitals of Morecambe Bay NHS Trust;
Honorary Consultant Paediatric and Adolescent Gynaecologist,
Royal Liverpool Children's Hospital

Mary Hernon MRCOG
Consultant Obstetrician and Gynaecologist,
Leighton Hospital, Crewe, Cheshire

Joanna Topping MRCOG
Consultant Obstetrician,
Liverpool Women's Hospital

Series Editor: Jenny Higham MD, FRCOG, FFFP, ILTM
Head of Undergraduate Medicine/Consultant Gynaecologist,
Faculty of Medicine, Imperial College London

BMA LIBRARY
BRITISH MEDICAL ASSOCIATION
WITHDRAWN FROM LIBRARY

RCOG PRESS

Published by the **RCOG Press**
at the Royal College of Obstetricians and Gynaecologists
27 Sussex Place, Regent's Park, London NW1 4RG

www.rcog.org.uk

Registered charity no. 213280

First published 2001; this edition 2008.

© 2008 The Royal College of Obstetricians and Gynaecologists

Apart from any fair dealing for the purposes of research or private study, criticism or review, as permitted under the Copyright, Designs and Patents Act, 1988, no part of this publication may be reproduced, stored or transmitted in any form or by any means, without the prior written permission of the publisher or, in the case of reprographic reproduction, in accordance with the terms of licences issued by the Copyright Licensing Agency in the UK. Enquiries concerning reproduction outside the terms stated here should be sent to the publisher at the UK address printed on this page.

The use of registered names, trademarks, etc. in this publication does not imply, even in the absence of a specific statement, that such names are exempt from the relevant laws and regulations and therefore for general use.

The publisher can give no guarantee for information about drug dosage and application thereof contained in this book. In every individual case the respective user must check its accuracy by consulting other pharmaceutical literature.

The rights of Anne Garden, Mary Hernon and Joanna Topping to be identified as Authors of this work have been asserted by them in accordance with the Copyright, Designs and Patents Act, 1988.

978-1-904752-58-5

Cover illustration: courtesy of Anne-Claude Juguet.

RCOG Editor: Jane Moody
Design/typesetting: Tony Crowley
Index: Liza Furnival, Medical Indexing Ltd
Printed in the UK by Latimer Trend & Company Limited, Estover Road, Plymouth, Devon PL6 7PY.

Contents

Preface

Paediatric and adolescent gynaecology adds an interesting dimension to the spectrum of work for gynaecologists but it can be intimidating, especially when one feels inadequately prepared. This concise book lays out the fundamentals of both investigation and management of the child and thereby enhancing confidence.

The text was extremely popular when the first edition was published and I have no doubt that this new edition will be equally successful. Professor Anne Garden is a recognised authority in this field and she has collaborated with colleagues to bring everything into contemporary focus. The new edition includes an important chapter on child sexual abuse – something a gynaecologist may encounter and has the obligation to do the right thing for the sake of the child.

The book is easy to read and makes a handy reference source for the MRCOG candidate and is also likely to be kept close at hand to refresh the memory of the established practitioner who intermittently encounters the younger patient.

Jenny Higham
Series Editor

Abbreviations

ACTH	adrenocorticotrophic hormone
BMI	body mass index
CAH	congenital adrenal hyperplasia
CAIS	complete androgen insensitivity syndrome
COCP	combined oral contraceptive pill
DHEAS	dehydroepiandrosterone sulphate
GnRH	gonadotrophin-releasing hormone
hCG	human chorionic gonadotrophin
HRT	hormone replacement therapy
LH	luteinising hormone
LSA	lichen sclerosus et atrophicus
MSH	melanocyte-stimulating hormone
PAIS	partial androgen insensitivity syndrome
PCOS	polycystic ovary syndrome
SD	standard deviation
SHBG	sex hormone-binding globulin
TDF	testis-determining factor

1 Pubertal growth and development

Menarche

The menarche is an important event in a girl's life and one that has special significance in many cultures. There has been a gradual reduction in the age of menarche in the UK over the 20th century, with a decrease of about 3–4 months per decade,[1] which has been thought to be due to improvements in health and nutrition. The average age of the menarche in 1840 was 16.5 years and is presently 12.8 years (with a normal range of 10.0–16.5 years). There has been a recent upturn in the age of menarche in the UK[2] for reasons that are not clear, although it has been suggested that an increase in exercise and the desire to be slim may be factors.[1] This reversal in the age of menarche has also occurred in other countries, including Iceland, Poland, Italy and Sweden but not Germany.

FACTORS DETERMINING THE AGE OF MENARCHE

Genetic factors
Nutritional factors
Socio-economic status
Geographic location
General health
Exercise

The age of menarche is determined by several factors. The importance of genetic factors is underlined by studies showing mother–daughter pairs and in twins, with identical twins having a closer relationship in age of menarche than non-identical twins.[3] The role of body weight and the percentage of body fat in the age of menarche has been debated, with the consensus of opinion being that weight is the more important factor. Girls who have a higher body mass index (BMI) in early childhood and a higher rate of change in BMI during childhood appear to undergo puberty earlier.[4] Girls who are heavier at the age of 7 years attain the menarche earlier than their peers,[5] a finding that also appears to be related to low birth weight. In the USA, the mean weight at menarche is 47.8 kg (SD ± 0.5 kg).[6] A study of 4427 girls, however, showed that relative weight for height at the age of 11 years accounted for only 5% of the variation in the age of menarche and concluded that the major influence was genetic.[7] Ninety-five percent of girls in the UK will have attained the menarche by the age of 15 years.

Endocrine basis of development, puberty and menarche

During fetal development, the hypothalamic–pituitary–ovarian axis is developed by mid-gestation. The high levels of estrogens produced by the placenta inhibit release of gonadotrophins from the pituitary. After delivery, with the withdrawal of these hormones, the levels of gonadotrophins increase, with some resultant ovarian activity; this may be sufficient to cause some neonatal breast development. The withdrawal of maternal hormones may also result in vaginal bleeding, which provokes real anxiety in the mother if she is not aware that this is may occur.

These effects do not last long, however, and within a short time of delivery, gonadotrophin levels drop and, thereafter, there is minimal gonadotrophin or ovarian activity throughout the years of childhood. Between the ages of 6 and 9 years, gonadotrophin levels gradually increase under the control of gonadotrophin-releasing hormone (GnRH) from the hypothalamus. GnRH is released in a pulsatile fashion, initially during sleep, and results in nocturnal augmentation of luteinising hormone (LH) secretion. As the duration of gonadotrophin release is prolonged, the ovary becomes more sensitive to its activity, with the stimulation of follicular growth and release of estrogens.

The final phase in pubertal development in endocrine terms is the development of the positive feedback mechanism by which the mid-cycle surge of gonadotrophins is produced.

Physiology of development, puberty and menarche

Under the influence of maternal hormones, the external genitalia of the neonate look well developed. The labia are large and rounded and often look quite oedematous; the hymen is thickened and prominent and a creamy white vaginal discharge may be present. With the loss of the maternal hormones, these appearances subside over the first few months of life, so that the labia majora become flattened, the labia minora become thin and attenuated and the hymen becomes less prominent. The hymenal changes take longer to occur so that, for the first year or so of life, it is not

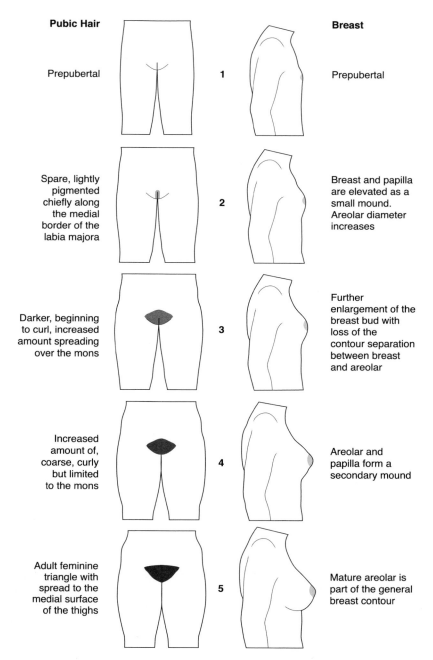

Pubic Hair

Prepubertal — 1 — Prepubertal

Spare, lightly pigmented chiefly along the medial border of the labia majora — 2 — Breast and papilla are elevated as a small mound. Areolar diameter increases

Darker, beginning to curl, increased amount spreading over the mons — 3 — Further enlargement of the breast bud with loss of the contour separation between breast and areolar

Increased amount of, coarse, curly but limited to the mons — 4 — Areolar and papilla form a secondary mound

Adult feminine triangle with spread to the medial surface of the thighs — 5 — Mature areolar is part of the general breast contour

Breast

Figure 1.1 Normal pubertal development (redrawn from Marshall and Tanner 1969, with permission)

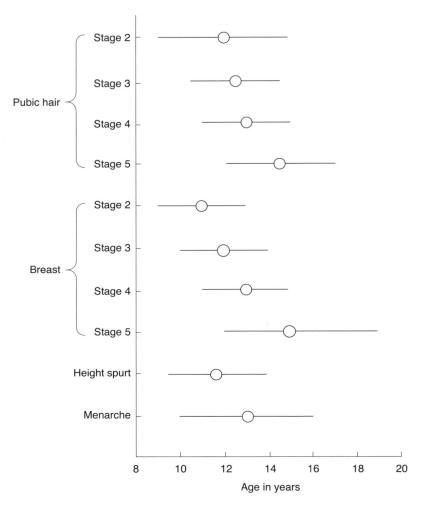

Figure 1.2 Age range for normal pubertal development in girls (redrawn from Marshall and Tanner 1969, with permission)

unusual for the hymen to appear as though it is prominent. The vaginal epithelium at birth is thick with numerous glycogen-containing cells within the squamous epithelium but, with the loss of maternal hormones, the epithelium becomes thin with loss of the glycogen-containing cells. In addition, the pH is raised and Döderlein's bacilli are absent.

The stages of pubertal development are described in the classic studies of Tanner and his colleagues in the 1960s and 1970s (Figures 1.1 and 1.2).

The first sign of puberty is the appearance of the sub-areolar breast bud at around the age of 10.8 years, with a normal range of 8.8–12.8 years. This is followed approximately 6 months later by early pubic hair growth, although in about one-third of girls pubic hair appears before the breast bud.[8] The increase in growth velocity closely follows the development of these early secondary sex characteristics but in some girls may precede them. Menarche usually occurs after this ordered sequence of pubertal development: spurt in skeletal growth; pubic hair development to Tanner stage 4 and breast development to Tanner stage 3–4.[9] The onset of menstruation is related to bone age, with 80% of girls reaching menarche at a bone age of 13–14 years and the remainder at a bone age of 12.5–14.5 years.[10] There is also a close relationship between growth velocity and menarche, with all girls starting to menstruate on the downward part of the growth velocity curve.

There is little growth in the size of the uterus up to the age of 9 years but growth occurs at Tanner stage 4, to about four times the prepubertal volume; by stage 5 it is five times larger.[8] The ovary remains fairly constant in size until the age of 5 years, when it begins to grow in relation to the girl's skeletal growth. A greater increase in the size of the ovary occurs with hormonal stimulus. Along with this increase in size comes an increase in follicular growth so that the ovary develops a multicystic appearance.

References

1. Rees M. Menarche when and why? *Lancet* 1993;342:1376–7.
2. Dann TC, Roberts DF. Menarcheal age in University of Warwick young women. *J Biosoc Sci* 1993;25:531–8.
3. Malina RM, Ryan RC, Bonci CM. Age at menarche in athletes and their mothers and sisters. *Ann Hum Biol* 1994;21:417–22.
4. Lee JM, Appugliese D, Kaciroti N, Corwyn RF, Bradley RH, Lumeng JC. Weight status in young girls and the onset of puberty. *Pediatrics* 2007;119:e624–30.
5. Cooper C, Kuh D, Egger P, Wadsworth M, Barker D. Childhood growth and age at menarche. *Br J Obstet Gynaecol* 1996;103:814–17.
6. Frisch RE. The right weight: body fat, menarche and ovulation. *Ballière's Clin Obstet Gynaecol* 1990;4:419–39.
7. Stark O, Peckham CS, Moynihan C. Weight and age at menarche. *Arch Dis Child* 1989;64:383–7.
8. Tanner JM. Puberty. In: Tanner JM. *Foetus into Man.* 2nd ed. Ware: Castlemead Publications; 1989. p. 58–74.
9. Marshall WA, Tanner JM. Variations in the pattern of pubertal changes in girls. *Arch Dis Child* 1969;44:944–54.
10. Marshall WA. Normal puberty. In: Brook CGD, editor. *Clinical Paediatric Endocrinology.* Oxford: Blackwell Scientific; 1981. p. 193–206.

2 Indeterminate genitalia

Many people believe that the management of children born with disorders of sexual differentiation is the major management problem in paediatric gynaecology. In fact, it forms only a small part of the practice of a paediatric gynaecologist, occurring in about one in 4500 births. The paediatric gynaecologist is but one member of the multidisciplinary team involved in the care of such children and their parents that includes a paediatric endocrinologist, neonatologist, paediatric surgeon, paediatric urologist, clinical geneticist, clinical psychologist and, if available, social work, nursing and medical ethicist.[1]

The first question asked by parents following delivery of their child is 'What sex is it?' Not to be able to answer that question is extremely distressing for all concerned and requires sensitive and informed care. Initial management should include giving the parents as full an explanation as possible but they should be warned that it may take some time before a complete answer can be given, although the information required to assign the sex of rearing is usually available within 48–72 hours.[2]

Embryological development

A degree of knowledge of the development of the internal and external genitalia is required to understand the clinical appearance of the child at birth. Chromosomal sex is determined at fertilisation and depends on whether the ovum is fertilised by a sperm bearing an X or a Y chromosome. Until about 6–7 weeks of gestation, the embryo develops in the same manner, irrespective of gender, and both sexes have both wolffian and müllerian ducts. After this, however, in the presence of a Y chromosome, the undifferentiated gonad develops into a testis. The absence of a Y chromosome results in the gonad developing into an ovary. In the presence of the testis-determining factor (TDF) containing the *SRY* (sex-determining region Y) gene on the Y chromosome, the germ cells are surrounded by Sertoli cells, which secrete anti-müllerian hormone, and the interstitial cells are differentiated into Leydig cells, which secrete testosterone under the stimulation of human chorionic gonadotrophin (hCG) from the placenta.

Testosterone begins to be secreted by the male embryo at around 8 weeks of gestation. This stimulates the wolffian ducts, causing the development of the epididymis, vas deferens and seminal vesicles. Conversion of testosterone to dihydrotestosterone by the enzyme 5-alpha reductase results in the development of the male urethra and prostate from the urogenital sinus and the external genitalia from the urogenital tubercle. The labioscrotal swellings fuse from the back to the front to form the scrotum. The anti-müllerian hormone secreted by the Sertoli cells causes degeneration of the müllerian ducts from about 9–11 weeks and, thus, suppression of the development of female internal genitalia.

Fetal pituitary gonadotrophin secretion begins in the fifth week of gestation but has a minimal contribution at that stage. It reaches a maximum by 20 weeks of gestation, however, and is responsible for the continued growth and development of the fetal testes. Development of the penis and scrotum are controlled by fetal LH and placental hCG, which are also responsible for descent of the testes.

In the absence of the Y chromosome, the supporting cells of the gonad become the granulosa cells that surround the oocytes, developed after meiotic division of the germ cells to form the primary follicles. Continued growth and development of the follicles is controlled by fetal pituitary gonadotrophins. The ovary, however, does not secrete a significant amount of estrogen, the vast majority of estrogen coming from the placenta.

Without anti-müllerian hormone, but not necessarily requiring the presence of an ovary, the müllerian duct develops into the fallopian tubes, uterus and upper two-thirds of the vagina. The wolffian ducts disappear in the female embryo. In the absence of dihydrotestosterone, the lower part of the vagina is formed from the urogenital sinus, the genital tubercle becomes the clitoris and the labioscrotal swellings remain separate to form the labia.

Causes of indeterminate genitalia

From the above, it can be seen that the development of the external genitalia is dependent on the presence or absence of androgens and not on the chromosomal or gonadal gender of the fetus. Previously, children with indeterminate genitalia were classified as 'intersex' but the term 'disorders of sexual differentiation' has been agreed.[3] The new classification is shown, together with the previous classification, in Table 2.1.

Irrespective of the cause, the clinical presentation is similar, owing to androgens acting on a female fetus or the insufficient action of androgens on a male fetus. The child has a phallus that is longer and wider than a normal clitoris but is not as large as a penis. The labia are fused to a varying degree, with a rugose appearance, and the urethral opening is usually on the perineum, at the base of the phallus, although it can be placed

Table 2.1   Classification of disorders of sexual differentiation (DSD)[3]

Previous	New	Causes
Female pseudohermaphrodite	46XX DSD	Congenital adrenal hyperplasia
Overvirilisation of an XX female		Iatrogenic
Masculinisation of an XX female		Androgen-secreting tumour
Male pseusdohermaphrodite	46XY DSD	Partial androgen insensitivity
Undervirilisation of an XY male		Mixed gonadal dysgenesis
Undermasculisation of an XY male		Poor androgen production
True hermaphrodite	Ovotesticular DSD	Unknown

anywhere on the ventral surface of the phallus or on the perineum anywhere on a line from the base of the phallus to the normal position of the female urethra. In a girl exposed to androgens, the degree of masculinisation depends on the gestation at which the exposure to androgens occurred,[4] as well as the level of androgens achieved in the fetus.

46XX disorders of sexual differentiation

CONGENITAL ADRENAL HYPERPLASIA

Congenital adrenal hyperplasia (CAH) is the most common cause of disorders of sexual differentiation and the most common cause of masculinisation of a female. CAH is a group of autosomal recessive disorders of adrenocortical steroid production caused by an abnormality in one of the group of enzymes involved in the conversion of cholesterol to cortisol. Of these, the most common is 21-hydroxylase deficiency, with an incidence of 1/5000–1/25000 in white populations.[5] The deficiency accounts for 95% of cases of CAH in the UK. Other enzyme deficiencies causing virilisation are 11-beta-hydroxylase and 3-beta-hydroxysteroid dehydrogenase. Their role in steroid production is shown in Figure 2.1. Deficiency of the enzyme leads to reduced production of the hormones distal to the block, accumulation of metabolites and abnormal production of hormones with unaffected production due to the feedback mechanism on adrenocorticotrophic hormone (ACTH) by the reduced cortisol production.

In the case of 21-hydroxylase deficiency, this translates into:

- reduction in the production of aldosterone (with resultant salt loss if the defect is also present in the zona glomerulosa) and of cortisol
- accumulation of 17-hydroxyprogesterone (the levels of which are used to monitor therapy)
- excess androgen production owing to the feedback mechanism.

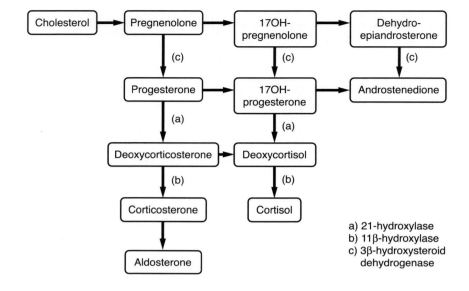

Figure 2.1 Algorithm of adrenal steroid production and the enzymes involved

The other enzyme disorders associated with CAH are beyond the scope of this book.

As the excess androgen production is present from conception, the degree of virilisation is usually marked and can be sufficiently severe that the girl is thought to be a normal male. There is marked phallic enlargement and labioscrotal fusion (Figure 2.2). Frequently, a urogenital sinus is present, resulting in a single perineal opening into which the urethra and vagina open at a higher level. The genitalia are frequently pigmented, owing to the increased production of melanocyte-stimulating hormone (MSH) together with ACTH from the anterior pituitary. Salt loss will be present in 50–75% of cases, causing dehydration and vomiting within a few days of birth and requiring urgent management. Antenatal therapy has been advocated because of the marked abnormality of the genitalia, with the necessity for major surgery in the neonatal period and possibly also at adolescence.

Prenatal diagnosis was first reported when a fetus, known to be female from prenatal karyotype studies, was thought to be male on ultrasound examination. DNA probes are now available that allow early detection before a major degree of virilisation has occurred. Treatment with maternal doses of dexamethasone will prevent the excessive fetal ACTH production.[6] There is, however, debate about the use of this treatment.

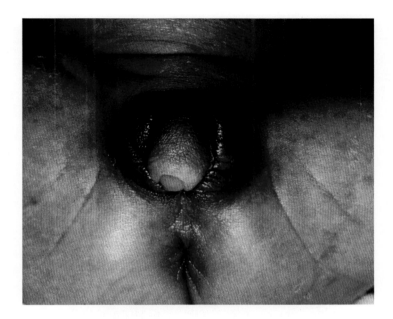

Figure 2.2 Indeterminate genitalia at birth in a child with congenital adrenal hyperplasia (courtesy of Parthenon Publishing)

IATROGENIC CAUSES

Iatrogenic causes of indeterminate genitalia are much less common and result from the prescribing of potentially masculinising drugs to the mother during the first 12 weeks of pregnancy. Such drugs include the C-19 nortestosterone-derived progestogens such as norethisterone or danazol, a 17-alpha ethinyl testosterone derivative. The degree of masculinisation is much less than in CAH, even in women who have taken the drugs throughout pregnancy, because the levels of androgen are much lower.

ANDROGEN-SECRETING TUMOUR

Virilising tumours of the maternal ovary or adrenal gland may cause masculinisation of the fetus but are extremely rare – particularly in pregnancy.

UNDERMASCULINISED MALE

Incomplete masculinisation of the wolffian ducts and external genitalia will also present with a complete spectrum of appearance of the genitalia, from a minor degree of hypospadias to apparently normal female genitalia.

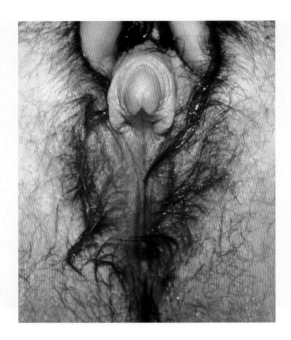

Figure 2.3 Virilised genitalia in an adolescent girl with partial androgen insensitivity (courtesy of Edward Arnold)

The condition results from either poor production of androgens by the fetus or from partial androgen receptor defects.

PARTIAL ANDROGEN INSENSITIVITY SYNDROME

Partial androgen insensitivity syndrome (PAIS), in common with the complete form of the receptor defect, (complete androgen insensitivity syndrome, see page 58) is an X-linked recessive disorder. It is caused by structural abnormalities of the androgen receptor gene as a result of point mutations resulting in alteration in androgen receptor messenger RNA or in single amino acids.[7] The phenotypic appearance is dependent on the degree of receptor defect. The child may have only a minor abnormality in appearance of the genitalia at birth, which becomes much more marked at puberty, owing to the higher levels of circulating androgens (Figure 2.3). Gynaecomastia may also occur at puberty.

MIXED GONADAL DYSGENESIS

Patients with gonadal dysgenesis (either 45X or 46XY) normally present as normal females with amenorrhoea. Patients with mosaic karyotypes

45X/46XY, 45X/47XYY or 45X/46XY/47XYY have been described, however. Such patients usually present with one palpable testis in the inguinal canal or in the scrotal sac. Hypospadias is usually present. Wolffian duct structures are present on the same side as the testis. The other side usually show a streak gonad, usually in the normal situation for an ovary, together with müllerian-duct derivatives and poorly developed wolffian structures.

POOR TESTOSTERONE PRODUCTION

Poor testosterone production can be caused by enzyme deficiencies or Leydig cell hypoplasia. The enzymes 3-beta-hydroxysteroid dehydrogenase, 17-alpha-hydroxylase and the cholesterol desmolase complex, as well as being involved in cortisol production, also have a role in androgen production. Other enzymes, including 17,20 desmolase and 17-beta-hydroxysteroid dehydrogenase, are purely involved in testosterone biosynthesis. 5-alpha-reductase is involved in the conversion of testosterone to dihydro-testosterone. This results in the genitalia appearing female at birth as, with the lack of dihydrotestosterone, there is poor penile development. Testes may be palpable in the labia. Internal genitalia, dependent on testosterone, are normal. The diagnosis may not be made until puberty when considerable, but not complete, virilisation may occur, together along with male psychosexual orientation. The penis remains small, however.

Management

As previously mentioned, psychological support for the parents is essential. They should be encouraged not to register the birth of the child or to decide a name for the child until the sex of rearing has been determined.

The appearance of the genitalia is not helpful in making a diagnosis but careful examination is required as part of the decision regarding the sex of rearing. Careful examination for the presence of gonads should be made. If both gonads are palpable, one of the forms of undermasculinised male is the likely diagnosis; hCG studies will help to differentiate between the various forms.

Decisions regarding the sex of rearing are made in consultation with the parents and depend on the appearance of the external genitalia and the likely functional outcome both for fertility and sexual relationships. Masculinised girls have potentially functioning ovaries and are potentially fertile. Reconstructive surgery is required, both to correct the appearance of the perineum and to open up the vagina from the urogenital sinus (Figure 2.4).

Undermasculinised males require investigation to assess the potential for penile growth and to maintain an erection. In addition, the testes are

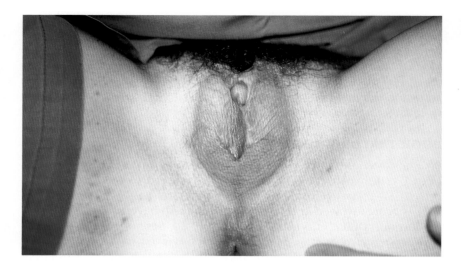

Figure 2.4 Adolescent girl with congenital adrenal hyperplasia prior to reconstructive surgery; clitoral reduction had been performed at birth; note the fused labioscrotal folds and single perineal opening

frequently abdominal and sufficiently high in the abdomen to make it difficult to bring them down while maintaining a blood supply. The testes will therefore have to be removed because of the risk of malignancy. This may affect the decision regarding the gender of rearing.

Surgery to reduce the clitoris must be performed with care to preserve the neurovascular bundle supplying the glans.[8]

Timing of surgery should also be discussed with the parents. For many parents, early reconstruction to achieve a normal appearance is important but surgeons prefer to wait until the child is older when there is more tissue to work with and the effects of estrogen make the tissues less friable. The finding that a higher incidence of sexual dysfunction is reported among girls who had early clitoral reduction surgery compared with those who had no surgery[9] has emphasised the importance of considering delaying such surgery until the girl herself is able to be part of the decision making process.

References

1. Lee PA. (2004) A perspective on the approach to the intersex child born with genital ambiguity. *J Pediatr Endocrinol Metab* 2004;17:133–40.
2. Meyers-Seifer CH, Charest NJ. Diagnosis and management of patients with ambiguous genitalia. *Semin Perinatol* 1992;16:332–9.

3. Hughes IA, Houk C, Ahmed SF, Lee PA, LWPES/ESPE Consensus Group. Consensus statement on management of intersex disorders. *Arch Dis Child* 2006;91:554–63.

4. Grumbach MM, Ducharme JR. The effects of androgens on fetal sexual development. Androgen induced female pseudohermaphroditism. *Fertil Steril* 1960;11:157–80.

5. Editorial. Congenital adrenal hyperplasia. *Lancet* 1987;ii:663–4.

6. New MI, Ghizzoni L, Speiser PW. Update on congenital adrenal hyperplasia. In: F. Lifshitz F, editor. *Pediatric Endocrinology.* New York: Marcel Dekker; 1996. p. 305–20.

7. Griffin JE. Androgen resistance – the clinical and molecular spectrum. *N Engl J Med* 1992;326:611–18.

8. Hutson JM, Voigt RM, Luthra M, Kelly JH, Fowler R. Girth reduction cliteroplasty – a new technique experience with 37 patients. *Pediatr Surg Int* 1991;6:336–40.

9. Minto CL, Liao LM, Woodhouse CR, Ransley PG, Creighton SM. The effect of clitoral surgery on sexual outcome in individuals who have intersex conditions with ambiguous genitalia: a cross-sectional study. *Lancet* 2003;361:1252–7.

3 Gynaecological conditions in childhood

Vaginal discharge is the only gynaecological condition that could be considered common in the prepubertal child and it is certainly the most common paediatric gynaecological problem presenting to the paediatric gynaecologist.[1] Other gynaecological problems seen in this age group include vulval irritation without discharge, labial adhesions and, occasionally, vaginal bleeding. Ambiguous genitalia, tumours and precocious puberty, although less common, warrant individual attention and are covered in the relevant chapters.

Vaginal discharge

The newborn female often has a clear or white odourless vaginal discharge, which is produced as a result of circulating maternal estrogen. Occasionally, in the neonatal period, the discharge may be bloodstained, owing to the breakdown of the endometrium, which has been stimulated by maternal estrogen levels.

As the child gets older, the most common cause of vaginal discharge is bacterial infection, commonly known as vulvovaginitis. Specific infections can occur in association with another focus of infection, such as a sore throat or a viral illness. The child transmits the infection from one part of the body to another digitally. This type of vulval infection causes few concerns, as it tends to resolve with the resolution of the primary infection. Recurrent non-specific infections, however, are difficult to manage. In the majority of cases, bacterial culture shows no growth or organisms of low virulence. Symptoms recur frequently, causing significant distress to both the child and parent, while proving difficult for the doctor to manage. This condition is known as recurrent bacterial vulvovaginitis.

RECURRENT BACTERIAL VULVOVAGINITIS

Recurrent bacterial vulvovaginitis is encountered most often in girls between the ages of 2 and 7 years and accounts for most cases of recurrent vaginal discharge.[2] This age range reflects the time when the mother ceases to supervise the perineal hygiene of her daughter as closely because the

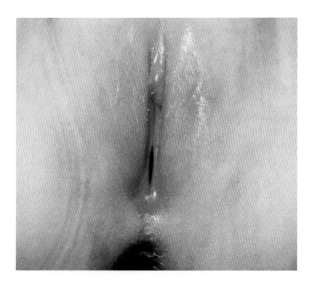

Figure 3.1 Normal prepubertal perineum showing flattened labia and the close proximity of the anus to the vagina

girl is now potty-trained. Girls may also start nursery or infant school, where the number of pupils makes careful supervision of toileting difficult. Thus, the young girl's attempts to keep herself clean are often inadequate.

The prepubescent girl also has an inherent susceptibility to vaginal infection, as she lacks the protective acid secretions of the older woman. In the newborn, the structure and physiology of the vagina and vulva are influenced by circulating maternal hormones. The vaginal epithelium is many layers thick, the cells are rich in glycogen and therefore the pH of the vagina is acid. Over the first few months the effects of maternal estrogen begin to decrease: the epithelium shrinks and the glycogen disappears. The pH of the vagina increases and it loses its natural acid protection. Thereafter, until estrogen levels increase at menarche, the vaginal mucosa is thin, atrophic and at increased risk of infection.

The anatomy of the perineum contributes to this increased risk. The vulval fat pads are poorly developed and the thin attenuated labia of a young girl flare outwards as she sits or squats and do not meet in the midline, thus exposing the vaginal opening and offering little protection from infection. The vaginal orifice is also in close proximity to the anus and at risk of soiling by faecal pathogens. The predilection of young children for sitting on the ground, grass or sand also increases contact with bacteria (Figure 3.1).

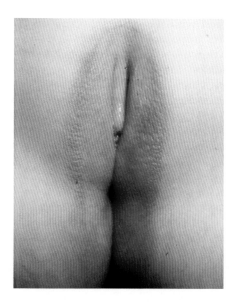

Figure 3.2 Vulval and perianal inflamation secondary to vulvovaginitis

PRESENTATION

The signs of recurrent bacterial vulvovaginitis are usually inflammation and discharge. Severity can vary dramatically and it is not unusual for there to be no abnormality at all on examination. It is therefore essential to obtain a good history from the parents. Not uncommonly, parents will present a history of recurrent offensive discharge, often green or yellow in colour, with associated significant pruritus or discomfort. The discomfort may be so severe as to prevent sleep or wake the child in the night. The skin irritation tends to cause scratching leading to excoriation. This may cause dysuria and can lead to an incorrect diagnosis of urinary tract infection. The symptoms seem to respond temporarily to treatment but invariably recur.

First presentation is usually after two or three episodes of vulvovaginitis. There may, however, be a delay of months, either owing to the parents' worry of allegations of abuse or secondary to a protracted period of self-medication with antifungal creams. This is usually because parents and health workers do not appreciate that candidiasis, so common in the baby and adult, is very rare in children.

When the young girl presents, a thorough inspection of the perineum for evidence of inflammation (Figure 3.2) should be undertaken and the child's underwear can be inspected to confirm the presence of discharge.

Examination is easiest with the girl supine and the legs in a frog-legged position. This allows inspection of the whole perineum. Often, young children will be worried about examination because of the significant discomfort this condition causes. An adequate inspection can be performed with the young girl lying supine on her mother's lap. Separation of the labia will allow the hymen to be inspected and a swab taken from the introitus. A small wire-tipped swab may be used if necessary.[3] The value of obtaining accurate identification of bacteria is debatable, as each new attack may be caused by a new infection and may involve a different organism or mixed growth.

We also have limited knowledge of the normal flora of the vagina of a prepubertal child. If an organism is cultured, the most common finding is group A beta-haemolytic streptococcus (*Streptococcus pyogenes*). In one study, there was a prior personal or family history of sore throat in over 50% of the patients.[4] *Haemophilus influenzae* is the next most commonly cultured pathogen. It was more common in the past but the Hib vaccination, introduced in 1985, is thought to be behind the decrease in number of cases. Staphylococci, coliforms and candida have also been isolated.[2] It is the strongly held belief of the authors that, if accurate bacteriological identification is necessary (as in cases of suspected abuse, which will involve taking swabs from above the hymen) this should be performed under general anaesthesia.

MANAGEMENT

There is no short answer or simple cure for recurrent vulvovaginitis. It is recommended that treatment with antibiotics only be initiated if there is pure or predominant growth of a pathogenic organism.[5]

Educating the parents and reassurance that the condition is self-limiting are vitally important. The basis for success is the understanding that each relapse is not due to the presence of a continuing infection but is a new infection. Parents have seldom felt able to discuss their daughter's condition with anybody and can feel isolated. Many parents present at a paediatric gynaecology clinic after repeated courses of antibiotics and a variety of creams, expecting that an examination under anaesthesia will give an answer for their daughter's problem. They are understandably upset to learn that this is not the case and it is important for the doctor to avoid examination under anaesthesia unless there has been bloodstained discharge or the discharge has failed to improve with conservative management.

The organisms responsible for recurrent bacterial vulvovaginitis tend to originate from the anus and nasopharynx or are picked up from the floor or grass where the child is sitting. Conservative management involves education on perineal hygiene and avoidance of risk factors. Advice given to parents and child should include advice on wiping the perineum from

Department of Surgery
Information for parents and carers
Vulvovaginitis

Introduction

Vulvovaginitis is a very common disorder that can affect females of all ages; it is one of the most common gynaecological conditions in school age children. This fact sheet aims to provide you with general information about this condition and suggestions to help deal with the condition.

What is it?

Vulvovaginitis is an inflammatory condition of the lower female genitalia.

What are the symptoms?

The main symptoms include a vaginal discharge, redness, soreness, itching and pain when passing urine.

Why is this happening?

Several factors are likely to make girls who have not yet reached puberty prone to this condition:
• Lack of the hormone estrogen, leads to a thin vaginal wall
• Lack of acidity in this area means that bacteria that is introduced can easily develop into an infection
• Children can easily transfer bacteria from their mouth ,nose and bottoms

Treatment

There is no standard treatment; occasionally girls will be given a course of antibiotics. Antibiotics will only deal with the current infection and will not prevent further infections.

What other treatments are available and what will happen if the condition is not treated?

Puberty will provide the body with the hormone estrogen and this will change the vaginal walls and turn a neutral environment to a more acidic environment; this enables the area to limit the effects of the bacteria and helps prevent further bacterial infections.

Factors to consider

While waiting for puberty, there are some factors to consider that may improve the current situation.
• Poor hygiene can introduce faecal bacteria so it is important that girls are taught to clean themselves thoroughly.
• Wearing loose fitting cotton underwear can be more comfortable.
• Avoid using perfumed soap, lotions, bubble bath and shampoo.
• Constipation, soiling and bed wetting are additional factors that need addressing by your GP, health visitor or school nurse.

Please contact your GP if you have any further concerns

This fact sheet gives only general information. You must always discuss the individual treatment of your child with the appropriate member of the hospital staff. Do not rely on this leaflet alone for information about your child's treatment.

This information can be made available in other languages and formats if requested.

Royal Liverpool Children's NHS Trust • Alder Hey • Eaton Road • Liverpool L12 2AP

Tel: 0151 228 4811
Web: **www.alderhey.com**

© RLC Alder Hey 2007

Figure 3.3 Patient information leaflet issued by Alder Hey Children's Hospital, giving advice on vulvovaginitis

front to back after going to the toilet and considering washing the perineum with soap and water after defecation. As vulvovaginitis appears to be more common in girls who are constipated, general dietary advice should be given. One study reported three cases where treatment of constipation was followed by resolution of the vulvovaginitis.[6]

Girls are encouraged to wear cotton underwear, to wear nightgowns rather than pyjamas and not to wear pants under their nightclothes. Tights, leggings and tight trousers are also discouraged. This involves a great deal of work by the parents and requires a great deal of tact from the doctor. If there is no evidence of poor hygiene contributing to the condition it is important to say so.

It is important to stress at all times that this is a self-limiting condition that will improve at the time of puberty and to ensure that both the girl and her parents are aware that there are no long-term complications of the condition. Parents often worry that recurrent infections may damage fertility or cause narrowing of the vagina.

If the discharge or irritation is particularly troublesome the best treatment is salt baths. Two large tablespoons of salt are added to a basin of water and the girl is encouraged to sit in it for about 10 minutes. The use of bland emollient creams such as zinc and castor oil can be used. These provide a barrier against further irritation from the discharge but can sting if the perineum is significantly inflamed. It is often useful to give an information leaflet to parents who bring their children to clinic with this problem (Figure 3.3).

If swabs from the vagina grow organisms associated with sexually transmitted infections, such as gonococcus, chlamydia or *Trichomonas vaginalis*, this is suggestive of sexual abuse and appropriate referral should be made according to NHS trust policy.[7] There is uncertainty regarding the significance of *Gardnerella vaginalis*. However, it is unusual in the absence of sexual activity and sexual abuse must be considered. It is important to remember that physical findings are only present in 4% of children who have been abused.[8]

There is no evidence that treatment with topical estrogen is of benefit in girls with recurrent vulvovaginitis.

Only if there is little significant improvement to symptoms after following instructions on perineal hygiene or there is any associated vaginal bleeding should the gynaecologist consider an examination under anaesthesia to be warranted, to exclude a foreign body.

Vulval irritation without discharge

The cause of vulval irritation without discharge is often difficult to diagnose. The main causes are threadworms, dermatological conditions and non-specific vulvitis.

THREADWORMS

Threadworms (*Enterobius vermicularis*) are extremely common in young children. Ova are excreted in the stools and transferred digitally across the perineum when the child scratches. Threadworms may also be found in the vagina. The classic symptoms are of perineal and vulval irritation, which tends to be worse at night when the adult worms emerge from the anus to lay their eggs. The diagnosis is made with the sticky tape test. A piece of sticky tape is applied to the perianal region at night and removed the following morning and attached to a glass slide. When viewed under the microscope adult worms and ova can be seen. The test does not have a good pick-up rate so it is possible to treat empirically if the symptoms are suggestive of infestation. Treatment is mebendazole 100 mg as a single dose. As the threadworms are easily transferred on toys or cups, all members of the family over 2 years of age should be treated.

DERMATOLOGICAL CONDITIONS

Any dermatological condition, such as eczema or psoriasis, can affect the perineal skin but these are seldom confined to that area and are not commonly seen by gynaecologists. Napkin rash is more specific to the

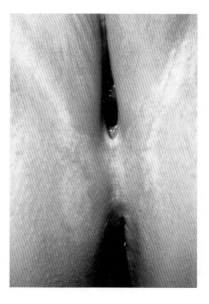

Figure 3.4 Mild lichen sclerosus demonstrating white plaques

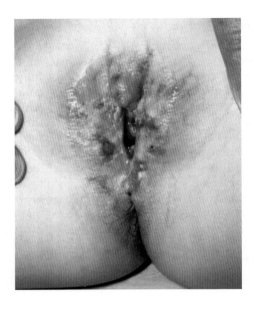

Figure 3.5 Severe lichen sclerosus showing ulceration and petechiae

perineum but tends to be managed in primary care; it is caused by wetting of the skin by urine and irritation from ammonia or possibly washing powder. Super infection with bacteria or candida is common. Treatment includes general advice about hygiene and the use of barrier creams to prevent further irritation.

LICHEN SCLEROSUS

Although not common, the dermatological condition most likely to be seen by a paediatric gynaecologist is lichen sclerosus et atrophicus (LSA). This is a chronic skin condition of unknown aetiology which appears to affect women at the extremes of life, being found most commonly in prepubertal girls and postmenopausal women. The incidence is difficult to estimate as a patient may present to many medical disciplines with lesions elsewhere on the body. Lichen sclerosus, however, has a strong predilection for the anogenital region.

The appearance is usually diagnostic, with irregular, shiny white macules or papules (Figure 3.4), which can coalesce into larger plaques. There are often associated areas of purpura and, in severe cases, alarming haemorrhagic bullae, erosions and ulceration (Figure 3.5). These lesions are caused by the increased fragility of the skin, not by excoriation. The dramatic appearance can lead to a mistaken diagnosis of sexual abuse unless the doctor is aware of the appearance of lichen sclerosus[9,10] and it has also been suggested that the condition is more common in children who have been abused.[11]

The girl presents with severe intractable irritation or discomfort, occasionally associated with bleeding. Vulval biopsy, mandatory in the postmenopausal sufferer, is usually not warranted in young girls, as the appearance is classical. If a biopsy is performed the histological features are of hypoplasia of the epidermis with flattening of the rete pegs. There may be hyperkeratosis on the surface of the epidermis with oedema and lymphocytic infiltration in the deeper dermis.

When the disease is mild or asymptomatic no treatment is required. Mild pruritus may warrant the use of a bland emollient. In severe cases the use of potent topical steroids is justified, such as clobetasol propionate 0.05%, applied twice daily for periods of up to 2 weeks. Most girls experience complete remission of their symptoms after 2 or 3 months of intermittent treatment and no maintenance therapy is required.[12] The prognosis for children with this disease is good and resolution may occur before puberty, although recurrence has been known.[13] Unlike LSA in the postmenopausal age group, there is no recognised risk of malignancy.

NON-SPECIFIC VULVITIS

Non-specific vulvitis is fairly common but is difficult to treat, as successful treatment depends upon identifying the precipitating factor and eliminating it from use. Common agents initiating or aggravating this condition include bubble-bath solutions, perfumed soap, washing powders (particularly biological ones) and fabric conditioners. Affected girls should wear loose cotton underwear, avoid wearing tight trousers or tights for any length of time and have their underclothes washed in a simple soap powder. Bland emollients may help as a barrier against irritation.

Labial adhesions

Adhesions are thought to be secondary to chronic irritation and are found most commonly in the toddler group. The young girls with labial adhesions appear to be relatively free of symptoms unless the adhesions are almost complete, which may lead to urine being trapped and the girl dribbling urine. The usual presentation is panic-stricken parents believing that their child has no vagina and usually wondering why they had not noticed this over the previous years. Inspection of the perineum easily differentiates labial adhesions from congenital absence of the vagina. In the former, the labia, clitoris, urethral meatus and hymenal orifice are easily visualised. In a child with labial adhesions, fused labia prevent visualisation of the hymenal ring, clitoris or urethral meatus. The adhesions form from back to front until

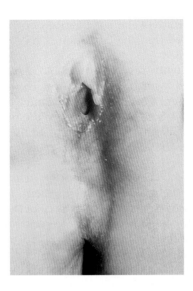

Figure 3.6 Labial adhesions involving the posterior part of the vulva (courtesy of Mark Allen Publishing)

only a small opening is left anteriorly (Figure 3.6). A fine translucent line can often be visualised along the line of fusion. Parents can be reassured that beneath the adhesions the child's anatomy is entirely normal.

If the girl is asymptomatic and the parents reassured by the explanation, diagnosis and the prognosis of spontaneous separation at puberty, no treatment is necessary. Treatment, if indicated, is simple: topical estrogen cream is applied twice daily along the line of fusion. This can either be carried out on a 2-week treatment/no treatment cycle, or used continuously, until separation occurs. Betamethasone cream 0.05% was a successful alternative to estrogen in one study.[14] Operative division is rarely warranted and should be reserved for patients who have not responded to medical treatment. As a risk of recurrence remains, even following surgery, it should be delayed until the girl approaches puberty to minimise the risk of recurrence.

Vaginal bleeding

Vaginal bleeding is a relatively unusual presenting symptom in a young girl. In the neonate it is likely to be secondary to the withdrawal of maternal estrogens. After the immediate neonatal period any vaginal bleeding requires serious investigation as a significant proportion may have some pathology.[15] Bleeding caused by precocious puberty and tumours are dealt with elsewhere in the book; the condition related to this chapter is the presence of foreign bodies.

Foreign bodies

Although the presence of a foreign body in the vagina should be considered when a child presents with an offensive or persistent vaginal discharge, this is relatively uncommon. In 200 girls presenting with vaginal discharge to the emergency room in a large children's hospital, foreign bodies were identified in only two and in these girls the discharge was bloodstained.[2]

The presence of blood staining in the discharge is highly suspicious of a foreign body. It is thought that bleeding is present in over 90% of cases where a foreign body is found.[16] If a foreign body is suspected, examination should be performed under anaesthesia. This is usually necessary when the child has a bloodstained discharge or a heavy discharge that is not improved by the use of conservative measures.[17]

The use of X-ray or ultrasound examinations to exclude foreign bodies in the vagina is not sufficient as plastic objects or tissue paper will not be seen. If examination under anaesthesia is being undertaken, a

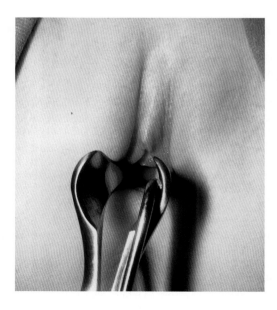

Figure 3.7 Use of nasal speculum to demonstrate foreign body

nasal speculum is commonly used for inspecting the vagina and cervix (Figure 3.7); other suitable instruments include a paediatric laryngoscope, cystoscope or a hysteroscope. It is important to continue inspection of the vagina as the instrument is withdrawn to ensure that no foreign body is missed.

Genital tract trauma

The most common genital tract injuries in this age group are straddle injuries caused by falling astride an object, commonly a fence or bicycle. The effect of such a fall is usually a painful haematoma of the labia. Treatment involves analgesia and the application of ice packs to reduce the swelling. If the haematoma continues to enlarge or is so painful that it is preventing micturition it may require drainage under anaesthesia. Tearing of the hymen or fourchette is not typical of a straddle injury and if a perineal haematoma is accompanied by either of the above injuries sexual abuse should be considered.

References

1. Huffman JW. Premenarchal vulvovaginitis. *Clin Obstet Gynecol* 1977;20,581–93.
2. Pierce AM, Hart CA. Vulvovaginitis: causes and management. *Arch Dis Child* 1992;67:509–12.
3. Hayes L, Creighton SM. Prepubertal vaginal discharge. *The Obstetrician & Gynaecologist* 2007;9:159–63.
4. Stricker T, Navratil F, Sennhauser FH. Vulvovaginitis in prepubertal girls. *Arch Dis Child* 2003;88:324–26.
5. Joishy M, Ashtekar CS, Jain A, Gonsalves R. Do we need to treat vulvovaginitis in prepubertal girls? *BMJ* 2005;330:186–8.
6. Van Neer PA, Korver CR. Constipation presenting as recurrent vulvovaginitis in prepubertal children. *J Am Acad Dermatol* 2000;43(4):718–19.
7. Thomas A, Forster G, Robinson A, Rogstad K; Clinical Effectiveness Group Association of Genitourinary Medicine; Medical Society for the Study of Venereal Diseases. National guideline for the management of suspected sexually transmitted infections in children and young people. *Arch Dis Child* 2003;88:303–11.
8. Johnson CF. Child sexual abuse. *Lancet* 2004;364:462–70.
9. Bays J, Jenny C. Genital and anal conditions confused with child sexual abuse trauma. *Am J Dis Child* 1990;144:1319–22.
10. Muhlendahl KE. Suspected sexual abuse in a 10-year-old girl. *Lancet* 1996;348:30.
11. Warrington SA, de San Lazaro C. Lichen sclerosis et atrophicus and sexual abuse. *Arch Dis Child* 1996;75:512–16.
12. Fischer G, Rogers M. Treatment of childhood vulvar lichen sclerosus with potent topical corticosteroid. *Pediatr Dermatol* 1997;14:235–8.

13. Berth-Jones J, Graham-Brown RAC, Burns DA. Lichen sclerosus. *Arch Dis Child* 1989;64:1204–6.

14. Myers JB, Sorenson CM, Wisner BP, Furness PD, Passamaneck M, Koyle MA. Betamethasone cream for the treatment of prepubertal labial adhesions. *J Pediatr Adolesc Gynecol* 2006;19:407–11.

15. Heller ME, Savage MO, Dewhurst J. Vaginal bleeding in childhood: a review of 51 patients. *Br J Obstet Gynaecol* 1978;85:721–5.

16. Paradise JE, English DW. Probability of vaginal foreign body in girls with genital complaints. *Am J Dis Child* 1985;139:472–6.

17. Smith YR, Berman DR, Quint EH. Premenarchal vaginal discharge: findings of procedures to rule out foreign bodies. *J Pediatr Adolesc Gynecol* 2002;15:227–30.

4 Endocrine disorders

Puberty is a dynamic continuum with the first signs in girls appearing at around the age of 9 years (see Chapter 1). Pubertal development that occurs before the age of 8 years is considered to be precocious. Precocious puberty occurs twelve times more commonly in girls than in boys. It may be central, in which there is premature activation of the hypo-thalamic–pituitary–ovarian axis or it may occur independent of the axis, in which case it is referred to as pseudopuberty or pseudosexual precocity.

Central precocious puberty

Central precocious puberty is also more common in females than in males by a factor of 23.[1] In girls, most causes are idiopathic (Figure 4.1). Causes identified include brain abnormalities, such as hydrocephalus, tumours

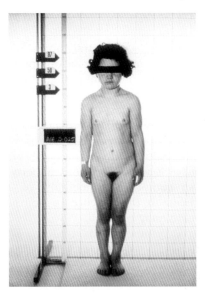

Figure 4.1 Precocious puberty in a five-year-old girl (courtesy of Parthenon Publishing)

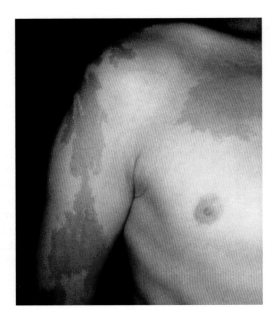

Figure 4.2 'Coast of Maine' appearance in a child with McCune-Albright syndrome (courtesy of Edward Arnold)

(particularly hamartomas), congenital abnormalities, trauma and infections. Hamartomas may cause precocious puberty at an extremely early age, even as early as the neonatal period. Precocious puberty is also associated with a wide variety of diverse conditions including neurofibromatosis, tuberous sclerosis and hypothyroidism. Hypothyroidism is particularly likely to be the diagnosis if the girl's pubertal development occurs without the accompanying growth spurt.

Because of the association with underlying brain pathology, it is recommended that all girls with precocious puberty have brain imaging performed with either computed tomography or, preferably, magnetic resonance imaging, even in the absence of neurological symptoms or signs,[2] as the abnormality may be small.

Girls with central precocious puberty undergo a normal sequence of pubertal development.

Pseudopuberty

Pseudopuberty is much less common than central precocious puberty and is characterised by raised estrogen levels in the absence of pubertal gonadotrophin levels. The most common cause is a hormone-secreting tumour such as a granulosa cell tumour or, less commonly, an arrhenoblastoma or thecoma.

A well-recognised but rare cause of pseudopuberty is the McCune–Albright syndrome.

PRESENTATION OF MCCUNE–ALBRIGHT SYNDROME

- characteristic areas of skin pigmentation, which can be fairly small, in the form of *café-au-lait* spots or larger areas often referred to as the 'coast of Maine' appearance (Figure 4.2)
- polyostotic fibrous dysplasia of the bone
- endocrine hyperfunction: gonadal activity most common form but thyroid, adrenal and pituitary activity also reported.

The cause of McCune–Albright syndrome is poorly understood but is thought to be a genetically determined signal transduction disorder. Mutations in the G-protein binding system stimulate production of the second messenger cyclic adenyl monophosphate, which causes autonomous hypersecretion of hormones.

Variations in pubertal development

Variations in pubertal development may also occur.

PREMATURE THELARCHE

Girls with this condition have premature isolated breast development, which may be bilateral or unilateral. The breast development may occur during the early years, often around the age of 2 years, and may fluctuate in appearance (Figure 4.3). There is no associated growth spurt and no development of pubic and axillary hair. Normal pubertal development is not affected nor is the girl's final height.

PREMATURE ADRENARCHE

Premature adrenarche is a common condition in which the girl develops pubic and axillary hair, often with associated sweat production. Girls who experience premature adrenarche are often overweight. There may be slight acceleration of growth and slight advance in bone age but this is not usually significant. Pubertal development is not otherwise affected. Care must be taken in these girls to exclude causes of excess androgen production, such as adrenal tumours, congenital adrenal hyperplasia and Cushing syndrome, in which cliteromagaly is often present.

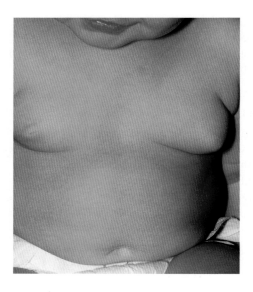

Figure 4.3 Premature thelarche in a girl of 18 months

PREMATURE MENARCHE

These girls present with isolated menstruation in the absence of pubertal development. Although the bleeding may be cyclical, they should be investigated as having abnormal vaginal bleeding an examination under anaesthesia should be performed, to exclude infection, tumour or trauma, as should an ultrasound examination to exclude an estrogen-secreting ovarian tumour. In addition, a hormone profile (including a GnRH stimulation test) should be performed.[3] Again, pubertal development is not usually affected.

Investigation of precocious puberty

Investigations should include estradiol and gonadotrophin estimations, thyroid function tests, ultrasound examination of the pelvis and X-ray of the wrist for bone age. If endocrine investigations confirm central precocious puberty, magnetic resonance imaging of the brain is indicated. If central precocious puberty is suspected but gonadotrophin levels are prepubertal, consideration should be given to performing a GnRH stimulation test. Levels of LH will be found to be raised to three of four times basal level in a girl with central precocious puberty compared with those found in a girl with pseudopuberty in whom gonadotrophin levels are suppressed.

Treatment of precocious puberty

The first decision to be made is whether or not the condition requires treatment. Factors that need to be considered include:

- age and maturity of the child
- rate at which the pubertal development is progressing
- psychological response of the girl to what is happening
- family situation.

A girl with marked pubertal development at the age of 3 years obviously requires treatment but a well-adjusted girl of 7 years with slow pubertal development, whose family are supportive and understand what is happening, may not require treatment.

The object of treatment is not just to stop pubertal development but also to ensure that her final adult height is not compromised. Adult height may be compromised not just because of early closure of the epiphyses but because the growth spurt occurs earlier in the child growth curve. For many girls and their families the paradox of a tall girl becoming a short adult is more difficult to deal with than the external signs of precocious development.

Treatment of central precocious puberty is with GnRH analogues. GnRH analogues will cause suppression of pubertal and skeletal growth and development, although it is not known whether final height prognosis is improved. There will be a reduction in uterine, ovarian and breast size, although there will not be a reduction in the size of the areola, which gives the breast a rather abnormal appearance, and the girl should be warned about this. Depending on the degree of endometrial stimulation that had occurred prior to treatment, a withdrawal bleed may also occur.

GnRH analogues are associated with weight gain but no other consistent adverse reactions and normal ovarian and menstrual function occur after therapy has been stopped,[4] although the number of girls treated remains small. There seems to be no long-term adverse effect on bone mineral density.[5]

In addition to treatment with GnRH analogues, it is important to give the girl and her parents full information about the mechanisms of puberty, the rationale for treatment and the limitations of treatment. They should be reassured that their daughter's puberty is abnormal in timing only and that treatment is only being used to control development until she becomes old enough to allow her development to continue.

Treatment of pseudopuberty

Treatment of pseudopuberty depends on the underlying cause. Obviously, underlying causes such as tumours require to be removed. Treatment of the gonadotrophin-independent forms of sexual precocity is with cyproterone acetate. This has been shown to suppress pubertal development but does not slow skeletal development and the prognosis for final height is not improved. Adverse effects include lethargy and excessive weight gain. Exaggerated adrenarche requires no intervention.

Most girls with precocious puberty have no subsequent problems in adulthood, although the fact that a minority do experience continuing problems has caused some researchers to suggest that all girls with precocious puberty should be followed up into adulthood.[6] There is no adverse effect on intelligence quotient or academic achievement.

Hirsutism

Hirsutism is defined as the presence of excessive facial hair in a female in a distribution that is characteristic of an adult male, owing to the effect of circulating free androgen levels on the hair follicles. It is an extremely embarrassing condition for any woman but particularly for a teenager.

Distribution of facial and body hair is race- and age-dependent. The amount of hair growth increases with age and is more obvious in such ethnic groups as those from the Indian subcontinent and from Mediterranean countries. Pathological causes of hirsutism include ovarian disorders, adrenal disorders, drugs and hypothyroidism (Figure 4.4). In many women, however, it is idiopathic. Of the identified causes, polycystic ovary syndrome (PCOS) is by far the most common, with late-onset adrenal hyperplasia the next most frequent.[7] Drugs associated with the development of hirsutism include androgen derivatives, such as danazol, and also non-androgenic agents such as phenytoin, corticosteroids and diazoxide.

As shown by the study quoted above, the most common identifiable cause of hirsutism in this age group is PCOS. This is discussed elsewhere (page 66). This disorder is characterised by hyperandrogenism and insulin resistance. The clinical presentation includes acne, irregular menstruation, obesity and infertility. The elevated LH levels found in those with PCOS cause increased levels of androstenedione and testosterone to be released by the ovary. This, together with the slightly low levels of sex hormone-binding globulin (SHBG) results in a higher level of free androgens causing hair follicle stimulation.

Late-onset congenital adrenal hyperplasia (CAH) is an autosomal recessive disorder which is particularly prevalent among Ashkenazy Jews. These girls usually present around puberty with increasing hirsutism and irregular periods. Diagnosis is achieved by measuring levels of 17-hydroxyprogesterone and androstenedione.

Any sign of virilism in association with the hirsutism is highly suggestive of an androgen-secreting tumour and should be investigated urgently.

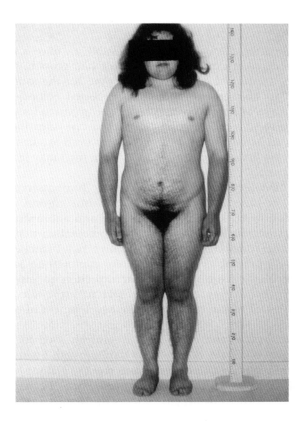

Figure 4.4 Hirsutism in a girl with Cushing syndrome (courtesy of Parthenon Publishing)

INVESTIGATION

Investigation of hirsutism should include careful examination of the whole body to document the degree of hirsutism, using a chart such as that described by Ferriman and Gallwey.[8]

Initial investigation of the cause is by hormone profile including FSH, LH, testosterone, SHBG, 17-hydroxyprogesterone and the specific adrenal androgen dehydroepiandrosterone sulphate (DHEAS). Cortisol, prolactin and thyroid function tests should also be carried out. If the girl is menstruating, LH and FSH levels should be assessed on day 2 of the cycle. Ultrasound scanning of the ovaries may also be helpful but a diagnosis of PCOS should not be made on ultrasound appearance alone. Further specific tests, particularly of adrenal function, may be required, depending on the initial screening results.

TREATMENT

Treatment should be started as soon as possible as, once a terminal hair follicle is stimulated, it can be difficult to stop hair growth. It should also be emphasised to the girl and her mother that, for the same reason, no improvement in hair growth should be expected before 6 months of treatment and a clear improvement may not be apparent for up to 2 years. Cosmetic treatment with waxing, electrolysis or sugaring should be considered as an adjunct to medical therapy or even as sole therapy if the condition is mild. Vaniqa® cream (Skin Medica, Inc.) may help in slowing regrowth of hair.

Treatment obviously depends on the cause. Tumours require surgical removal and late-onset CAH is treated with hydrocortisone.

Hirsutism due to PCOS is treated with the anti-androgen cyproterone acetate in conjunction with estrogen. This combination may be given in the form of the combined oral contraceptive pill Dianette® (Schering Health; ethinyl estradiol 35 micrograms and cyproterone acetate 2 mg). Estrogen is necessary to ensure regular menstruation, to raise the levels of SHBG and so reduce free testosterone and to prevent conception, as cyproterone acetate will interfere with the development of male genitalia in a male fetus.

Cyproterone acetate and estrogen may also be used in the reversed sequential regimen initially described by Hammerstein,[9] with cyproterone acetate 50–100 mg daily being given from day 5–14 along with Dianette from day 5–25. Once hair growth is controlled, it may be maintained with a lower dose of cyproterone acetate, often with Dianette.

Adverse effects of cyproterone acetate include tiredness, excessive weight gain and, rarely, adrenal suppression. Hepatotoxicity has been reported and liver function tests should be performed at 6-monthly intervals when on the higher dose. Different approaches are used to manage the problem. Some clinicians prefer to start with the higher-dose regimen of cyproterone acetate, to obtain maximum effect on hair growth, and to change to Dianette for maintenance. Others prefer to use the lower dose of cyproterone acetate in Dianette in the first instance in order to minimise the adverse effects of the drug, changing over to the higher-dose treatment if there is no response. It is a difficult decision, particularly in this age group, in whom appearance is so important. The decision should be made in conjunction with the girl in order to maximise compliance.

Although its main use has been in the management of infertility, increasingly, metformin has been used in the treatment of teenagers with PCOS. Although less effective than the combined oral contraceptive pill, it has been shown to be effective in the regulation of menstruation and in the reduction of serum androgen levels. It also lowers fasting insulin levels and triglyceride levels.[10] The main adverse effects of metformin levels are gastrointestinal – nausea, bloating and diarrhoea. These can be minimised by slowly increasing the dose of metformin and advising that it be taken with meals. Girls on metformin therapy should have their renal and liver function checked regularly.

Although not licensed in the UK for this indication, spironolactone has been used successfully in the treatment of hirsutism.[11]

Virilism

Virilism is rare but potentially serious. In addition to hirsutism, clitoral hypertrophy, male-pattern baldness, breast atrophy and deepening of the voice may all be present. Virilism is caused by excess androgen production, the common causes being an androgen-secreting tumour, either from the ovary or the adrenal gland, CAH, Cushing syndrome and PAIS. In an adolescent, PAIS and CAH are the most common, with androgen-secreting tumour being the most serious.

Investigations include testosterone, androstenedione, DHEAS, cortisol, ACTH and 17-hydroxyprogesterone. Twenty-four-hour urinary steroid profiles are particularly helpful. Ultrasound scanning of the ovaries and magnetic resonance imaging of the adrenal gland should be performed if investigations suggest a tumour. The treatment is dependent upon the cause.

References

1. Bridges NA, Christopher JA, Hindmarsh PC, Brook CG. Sexual precocity, sex incidence and aetiology. *Arch Dis Child* 1994;70:116–18.

2. Kornreich L, Horev G, Blaser S, Daneman D, Kanli R, Grunebaum M. Central precocious puberty, evaluation by neuro-imaging. *Paediatr Radiol* 1995;25:7–11.

3. Pinto S, Garden A. Pre-pubertal menarche: a defined clinical entity. *Am J Obstet Gynecol* 2006;195:327–9.

4. Jay N, Mansfield MJ, Blizzard RM, Crowley WF Jr, Schoenfeld D, Rhubin L, Boepple PA. Ovulation and menstrual function of adolescent girls with central precocious puberty after therapy with gonadotrophin releasing hormone agonists. *J Clin Endocrinol Metab* 1992;75:890–4.

5. Neely EK, Bachrach LK, Hintz RL, Habiby RL, Slemenda CW, Feezle L, *et al.* Bone mineral density during the treatment of central precocious puberty. *J Pediatr* 1995;127:819–22.

6. Rosenfield RL. Normal and almost normal precocious variations in pubertal development, premature pubarche and premature thelarche revisited. *Horm Res* 1994;41 Suppl 2:7–13.

7. Baron JJ, Baron J. Differential diagnosis of hirsutism in girls between 15 and 19 years old. *Ginekol Pol* 1993;64:267–9.

8. Ferriman D, Gallwey JD. Clinical assessment of body hair growth in women. *J Clin Endocrinol Metab* 1961;21:1440–7.

9. Hammerstein J. Possibilities and limits of endocrine therapy. In: Hammerstien J, Lachnit-Fixson U, Neumann F, Plewig G, editors. *Androgenisation in Women.* Amsterdam: Excerpta Medica; 1980. p. 221–34.

10. Costello M, Shrestha B, Eden J, Sjoblom P, Johnson N. Insulin-sensitising drugs versus the combined oral contraceptive pill for hirsutism, acne and risk of diabetes, cardiovascular disease, and endometrial cancer in polycystic ovary syndrome. *Cochrane Database Syst Rev* 2007;24(1):CD005552.

11. Erenus M, Yuceltin D, Gurbaz O, Durmusoglu F, Pekin S. Comparison of spironolactone-oral contraceptive versus cyproterone acetate-estrogen regimens in the treatment of hirsutism. *Fertil Steril* 1996;66:216–19.

5 Child sexual abuse

Child abuse has existed for centuries but society has been slow to acknowledge it. It can constitute physical, emotional and sexual abuse as well as neglect. Up until the 17th century, children were considered to be the possessions of their parents and it was accepted that they might harm them. It was only in the 1970s that non-accidental injury of children was accepted as a common occurrence, following the description of battered child syndrome in 1962. Corporal punishment existed in schools in Britain until 30 years ago and was thought to be a necessity. Now there is debate regarding the smacking of children.

The first child protection agency was formed in Liverpool in 1883, followed by the National Society for the Prevention of Cruelty to Children (NSPCC) in 1890. The start of the education system in 1870 allowed for children to be observed at school every day for the first time.

Child sexual abuse was less talked about. Incest was a crime according to the Christian Church from the 1700s but was only made a criminal offence in the UK in 1908. Papers in the literature relating to child sexual abuse start mainly from the 1980s. There have been many high-profile cases reported in the press over the years, such as Maria Colwell in 1974, the Cleveland Inquiry in 1987 and, more recently, Victoria Climbie, who died in 2000 with 108 injuries on her body. All have highlighted loopholes in the child protection system. Close cooperation between social services, the police and healthcare professionals is imperative. Recognition, communication, knowledge of child protection procedures and note keeping are key factors in all enquiries.

What is it?

The definition of physical abuse has altered over the years with society, culture and views on corporal punishment. It is still debated and likely to evolve. However, all types of sexual abuse involve the use of a child below the legal age of consent for the sexual gratification of an adult or significantly older child.[1] This definition is taken from *Working Together to Safeguard Children.*[2]

Abuse and neglect are forms of maltreatment of a child. Somebody may abuse or neglect a child by inflicting harm or by failing to act to prevent harm. Children may be abused in a family or in an institutional or community setting; by those known to them or, more rarely, by a stranger. They may be abused by an adult or adults or another child or children.

Sexual abuse involves forcing or enticing a child or young person to take part in sexual activities, including prostitution, whether or not the child is aware of what is happening. The activities may involve physical contact, including penetrative (for example, rape, buggery or oral sex) or non-penetrative acts. They may include non-contact activities, such as involving children in looking at, or the production of, pornographic material or watching sexual activities, or encouraging children to behave in sexually inappropriate ways.

Physical and emotional abuse and neglect have separate definitions. They frequently occur concurrently.

Who are the victims?

A national survey of young people by the NSPCC, published in 2000, reported a prevalence of sexual abuse of 16%.[3] Depending on the population studied and the definition of child sexual abuse, 2–62% of women and 3–16 % of men have been abused.[1]

There is no doubt that there has been a significant increase in reported cases in the last decade of the 20th century. There is greater public awareness of the subject, children are taken seriously when they voice their concerns and independent agencies have been set up, such as 'Childline', where children can obtain confidential advice. The exact extent of child sexual abuse is not known. Much abuse occurs within families and there is therefore tremendous pressure not to disclose.

Children of all ages and backgrounds can be abused but there are identifiable risk factors.[3] The factors associated with sexual and other types of abuse are difficult to separate:

- child factors
- parental factors
- environmental factors.

The child is more likely to be abused if he or she was unwanted, owing to failure to meet expectations, breakdown of parents' relationship, being progeny of forced sex or prostitution, if there were long periods of separation from the parent, such as hospitalisation, if the child has disabilities, behavioural problems, prolonged soiling, wetting or crying beyond developmental age.

Parental factors include presence of step-parents, teenage, single or disabled parents, antisocial personality, drug or alcohol abuse, mental health problems, being abused themselves as a child, many children with less than 18 months between births, domestic violence and importantly, previous record of sexual offences. Environmental factors include poor housing and neighbourhood, family violence, violence to pets, social isolation and poverty.

Interviews with perpetrators in custody revealed a tendency to seek attractive children from single-parent families with low self-esteem and low confidence who were easily manipulated and lonely. They found their victims in playgrounds, at family events and near their homes and abused them in the perpetrator's or the child's home. They 'groomed' the children with play, gifts and understanding. They used techniques to 'disinhibit' children involving drugs, alcohol and pornography then maintained the relationships with threats of hitting and hurting the victims or their loved ones.[1]

Who are the abusers?

The vast majority of perpetrators of sexual abuse on children are male. There are no distinguishing features for people who abuse children: they come from all social classes and cultural backgrounds. They are usually known to the victim: a relative or male member of the household (mother's boyfriend) or a temporary carer. It is common for abusers, when discovered, to leave but move to a new relationship within a household of similar composition so that abuse can continue.

Presentation

A child who is being sexually abused may present to a multitude of different agencies or medical disciplines. Disclosure of an allegation of abuse may be made by the child to the doctor or another professional. The onus is then on the doctor to take further action. It is important that the child is taken seriously. If the child has disclosed the identity of the abuser, a return home may expose the child to significant risk of reabuse, physical harm or pressure to change their story. The doctor should inform the police or social services department promptly, with the knowledge of the carer.

Child sexual abuse should be remembered in the differential diagnosis of many conditions. Those that are likely to be seen by a gynaecologist include:

- genital soreness
- genitourinary injuries, such as vaginal bleeding laceration or bruising
- discharge
- recurrent dysuria in the absence of proven urinary tract infections
- sexually transmitted infection
- pregnancy, especially when the identity of the father is withheld
- request for termination of pregnancy.

Other physical symptoms include faecal soiling, retention or rectal bleeding, a return of enuresis and nonspecific abdominal pain. It is possible that a child may present to hospital for one problem and, on examination, be found to have injuries that are not consistent with the history.

The occurrence of certain types of behaviour patterns may suggest that a child is being abused. These include:

- inappropriate sexual behaviour
- self-harm
- eating and sleeping disorders
- under-achieving.

Children may be victims of more than one form of abuse. This must be borne in mind when dealing with children presenting with evidence of non-accidental injury or emotional abuse and neglect. In any case where child sexual abuse is suspected a full history must be taken. This will help the doctor decide whether abuse is probable or a possibility.

History

The history should include a description of the alleged events, including discomfort or bleeding. Was there a history of kissing or licking (swabs can be taken for DNA typing from saliva)? Specific details of the abuse, when volunteered, should be written in the words of the child. A full paediatric history needs to be obtained, with special attention being paid to any history of vulval irritation, dysuria or bowel dysfunction. If the victim is an adolescent, a menstrual history should be taken, to include type of sanitary protection used (pads or tampons), number of boyfriends and any history of sexual intercourse or digital exploration. Any history of straddle injuries should be elicited and whether the child has ever experimented with or been offered alcohol or drugs.

If the history of abuse is uncertain in that the statement by the child is vague or symptoms nonspecific, a thorough physical examination of the child, including inspection of the anogenital area, should be undertaken.

The case should be discussed with senior colleagues or other agencies, as there may be other areas of concern known to health visitors or social workers. A family history of concern may be known to the GP but not to a hospital doctor. Follow-up should be arranged.

Examination

Although doctors should be aware that the probability of finding definite clinical evidence of abuse is low, the performance of a thorough examination is important for several reasons:[4]

- the possibility of obtaining forensic samples, which can be used if a prosecution is undertaken
- the need to treat any injuries or infections the child may have
- a thorough examination will allow the doctor to reassure the child and family that no long-term physical damage has occurred.

This reassurance allows the first step in the healing process to occur.

TIMING OF EXAMINATION

There is rarely a need for immediate examination by the attending doctor unless the child has an injury or condition requiring immediate attention. It is more important that the person performing the examination is skilled in paediatric examination and has knowledge of normal genital and anal anatomy in prepubescent children. If the alleged assault is recent, the child should not be bathed or change her clothes before the examination. Most positive forensic findings were found in children seen within 72 hours in one study at a specialist referral centre.[5]

In many areas, police surgeons or forensic medical examiners and paediatricians work in close cooperation, allowing a single examination to be used to look for confirmatory signs and collect evidence such as samples or photographs. The performance of numerous examinations is disturbing and compounds any abuse to which the child has already been subjected.

PLACE OF EXAMINATION

Wherever possible, the examination should be carried out away from the formal and busy clinical setting, preferably in specially designed suites that are less intimidating for the child. Often a colposcope is available, which offers good illumination and magnification of the genital area and allows photographs or video to be taken by the attending doctor. Otherwise, some form of medical photography needs to be readily available.

PERFORMING THE EXAMINATION

Any examination can only be done with the child's consent. The Children Act 1989 gives young people the right to decline examination. The quality of examination one can perform on an uncooperative child is debatable and the psychological trauma can only compound the initial abuse.

The child should not be examined without the knowledge and agreement of a parent. The name of the person with parental responsibility should be recorded in the notes along with a signed consent form. If the history is suggestive of abuse and the parent will not give consent for examination, it is necessary to obtain consent from the court. This should be arranged in consultation with the social services and police, by means of an emergency protection order. The mother should be present, if possible, at the examination of any prepubescent child. Adolescents should be given the option of having somebody present.

A general physical examination should be undertaken, including height and weight, as children subject to any form of abuse often fail to thrive. The general examination should continue with inspection of the eyes, mouth, chest and abdomen. Not only will this reveal evidence of bruising but it will give the child time to relax so that examination of the genitalia and anus become a routine part of the procedure.

Often, nothing more than inspection of the genitalia is required, using a colposcope to illuminate and magnify the area. If the alleged abuse has occurred within the last 72 hours it may be possible to obtain forensic samples of semen or blood to allow DNA identification. These should be collected using appropriate sexual offences kits provided by police or forensic laboratories. It is also important to take samples for sexually transmitted infections, including first-catch urine for chlamydia and gonococcus, swabs for or *Trichomonas vaginalis* infection and other potentially sexually transmitted organisms. This should be done in conjunction with a genitourinary medicine department and according to

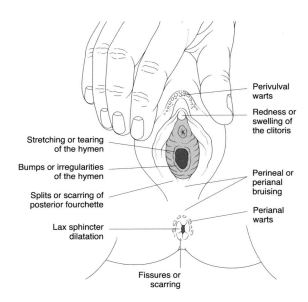

Figure 5.1 Genital and anal findings that may indicate abuse

national guidelines.[6] The only test currently recognised in court for evidential purposes for chlamydia, gonococcus and *T. vaginalis* is culture, despite many laboratories not now offering this test and its suboptimal sensitivity. This is under review. The incubation period of sexually transmitted infections and the timing of serological tests for HIV and hepatitis B mean that follow up by a genitourinary medicine department is essential. Post-exposure prophylaxis for HIV and vaccination for hepatitis B are not evaluated in children but may be considered. The girl may need emergency contraception.

The anogenital examination is usually carried out with the child supine on a couch in the frog-legged position. The labia should be parted by the examiner to allow inspection of the introitus and hymen. However, in this position, the posterior part of the hymen may not be visualised; the use of a Foley catheter inserted into the vagina then the balloon inflated and gently withdrawn will usually allow this to be achieved. The posterior aspect of the hymen can often be more easily demonstrated in the knee–chest position but if the child has been subjected to any form of anal abuse this can be too traumatic. Inspection of the anus is easiest in the left-lateral position. If the child is young enough and would prefer it, a satisfactory examination can be conducted with the child lying on her mother's knee.

Findings

It must be stressed that the absence of abnormal findings does not refute the diagnosis of sexual abuse.[7] In 2384 children referred for possible child sexual abuse, only 4% had abnormal genital or anal examinations.[8] Some forms of abuse, such as touching and licking and viewing pornography, may not produce physical findings. It is also important to remember that, at the present time, there is no single diagnostic test available. It is therefore paramount that all information is clearly documented, preferably with the aid of diagrams and photographs (Figure 5.1).

General examination may reveal bruising consistent with the child having been forcibly held; this may be evident on the arms or possibly on the inner thighs.

APPEARANCE OF THE HYMEN

In most children, the hymen is a smooth, elastic membrane with a smooth-edged opening. It is important to spend some time observing the hymen. A hymen may open up as a child relaxes, revealing healed tears or bumps (Figure 5.2). Its appearance varies with the age of the child and the position in which the child is examined. Some dents and bumps, although considered to be suspicious in the past, have been found to be normal.[1]

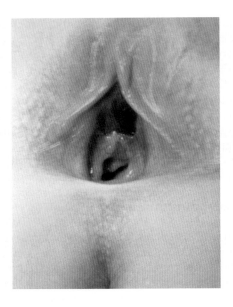

Figure 5.2 Anterior notch in hymen indicating old tear

Findings considered to be suspicious of penetration are a significant increase in the transverse diameter of the hymen (although there is a significant overlap with normal diameter so this is not a diagnostic sign), narrowing of the posterior rim of the hymen to less than 1 mm and complete hymenal clefts between the 5 o'clock and 7 o'clock positions. The hymen usually tears on the posterior aspect. Tears can heal completely in a very short time or can leave clefts or V-shaped notches which approach the vaginal floor. If the hymen cannot be seen easily, a Foley catheter may be required to facilitate examination.

APPEARANCE OF LABIA AND FOURCHETTE

There may be reddening or bruising of the labia in cases of acute abuse. There may also be reddening or bruising of the vulva and tears or old scars at the fourchette. Occasionally, labial adhesions may be found. Labial adhesions are caused by chronic irritation and therefore repeated abuse may contribute to their formation. Perineal bruising or bleeding may be noted and the presence of dilated veins.

Inspection of the anus may demonstrate no abnormality or signs of abuse, such as the presence of deep fissures crossing the anal skin margin; scars or skin tags may be left from old injuries. Some forms of penetration may result in damage to the internal anal sphincter resulting in 'reflex' anal dilatation when the child is observed in the left-lateral position with the buttocks parted for 30 seconds. This sign is of limited value as, if a child lies in the frog-legged position for any length of time, the anus will pout. Indeed, this can be a consequence of the passage of large stools as a result of constipation, so is not diagnostic. The sphincter will also lose tone under general anaesthesia.

The findings of examinations performed when sexual abuse is an issue, together with photographs and videocolposcopy, should be discussed and reviewed with medical peers involved in child protection, as this minimises errors. It is important to remember than many children who have never been abused can show atypical appearances in the anogenital area[9,10] and that an abnormal finding with no history suggestive of abuse is most likely to be due to an alternative condition rather than abuse.

Long-term consequences and follow-up

In the past, health professionals concentrated solely on identification of and protection of children from sexual abuse. Realisation of the long-term effects resulted in the introduction of intervention therapies. The psychological effects of sexual abuse can be severe and prolonged into adulthood. They include anxiety and depression, eating disorders, post-traumatic stress disorder and suicide. Pregnancy and HIV result in lifelong effects. There is evidence of the 'victim to victimiser' cycle, whereby children who were sexually abused become abusers themselves. It must be stressed that this only happens in a minority of victims, who are usually male, and is more common when the abuser was female.[11]

Referral for psychological assessment and support should therefore be part of the routine follow-up of abused children. The doctor should always arrange emergency contraception or a pregnancy test if indicated. Gynaecological follow-up may be of benefit to check the healing of any areas of trauma and ensure that any infections found at initial examination have been treated adequately. Genitourinary medicine follow-up has been mentioned already.

When a doctor undertakes to examine a child for alleged sexual abuse, they must be prepared to present their findings at case conferences and possibly court proceedings. It is therefore essential that all case notes be made scrupulously with this eventuality in mind.

Prevention

Prevention education of children throughout their school life and of their parents is thought to be of value. Television viewing and internet usage by children should be monitored by parents. In the USA, parents are made aware of the location of paedophiles in their communities.

Doctors must be able to recognise and report child sexual abuse and understand that this is an effective means of prevention of further abuse (in childhood or adulthood) and reactive abuse. The children and the perpetrators should receive treatment.

The effects of sexual abuse can be long-term and life-threatening. It affects the victims, their families, their future partners and society as a whole. Gynaecologists, in particular, should have a high awareness of both the existence of child sexual abuse and its association with many gynaecological conditions in the child or the adult.

References

1. Johnson CF. Child sexual abuse. *Lancet* 2004;364:462–70.

2. HM Government. *Working Together to Safeguard Children: A guide to inter-agency working to safeguard and promote the welfare of children*. London: The Stationery Office; 2006 [www.everychildmatters.gov.uk/resources-and-practice/IG00060/].

3. Polnay J, Polnay L. *Child Protection Reader: recognition and response in child protection*. London: Royal College of Paediatrics and Child Health; 2006 [www.rcpch.ac.uk/Health-Services/Child-Protection/Child-Protection-Publications].

4. Bamford F, Roberts R. Child sexual abuse – II. In: Meadows R, editor. *ABC of Child Abuse*. 3rd ed. London: BMJ Publishing Group; 1997. p. 40–6.

5. Palusci VJ, Cox EO, Shatz EM, Schultz JM. Urgent medical assessment after child sexual abuse. *Child Abuse Negl* 2006;30: 367–80.

6. Thomas A, Forster G, Robinson A, Rogstad K; Clinical Effectiveness Group Association of Genitourinary Medicine; Medical Society for the Study of Venereal Diseases. National guideline for the management of suspected sexually transmitted infections in children and young people. *Arch Dis Child* 2003;88: 303–11.

7. Bays J, Chadwick D. Medical diagnosis of the sexually abused child. *Child Abuse Negl* 1993;17:91–110.

8. Heger A, Ticson L, Velasquez D, Bernier R. Children referred for possible sexual abuse: medical findings in 2384 children. *Child Abuse Negl* 2002;26:645–59.

9. McCann J, Wells R, Simon M, Voris J. Genital findings in prepubertal girls selected for non-abuse. *Pediatrics* 1990;86:428–39.

10. Kellog ND, Parra JM, Menard S. Children with anogenital signs and symptoms referred for sexual abuse evaluations. *Arch Pediatr Adolesc Med* 1998;152:634–41.

11. Glasser M, Kolvin I, Campbell D, Glasser A, Leitch I, Farrelly S. Cycle of child sexual abuse: links between being a victim and becoming a perpetrator. *Br J Psychiatry* 2001;179:482–94.

6 Amenorrhoea

Amenorrhoea is not as common a problem as heavy and painful periods but is often poorly understood and managed. Amenorrhoea is a symptom that requires investigation and not a diagnosis in itself.

> **AMENORRHOEA**
>
> **Primary:** girl has never experienced a menstrual period
> **Secondary:** periods have been absent for 6 months or more.

Causes of primary amenorrhoea

The causes of primary amenorrhoea are considered differently, depending on whether or not secondary sexual characteristics are present (Figure 6.1). In girls with no secondary sexual characteristics, the cause is usually hormonal, whereas in girls with normal pubertal development the cause is usually anatomical.

As a general rule, girls who have primary amenorrhoea with no secondary sexual characteristics should be investigated by the age of 14 years. Common causes include:

- constitutional delay
- chronic systemic disease
- absence of ovarian function
- hypothalamic pituitary dysfunction.

CONSTITUTIONAL DELAY

These girls have delayed maturation of the hypothalamic–pituitary–ovarian axis, with resultant delay in the whole process of puberty. There is frequently a family history of similar symptoms in the mother or older siblings. Examination shows a normal relationship between skeletal growth and sexual maturity. Hormone profile shows low levels of FSH, LH and estradiol. Estimation of bone age, if performed, will show delayed skeletal maturation with the bone age being behind the chronological age. Ultrasound examination of the ovaries may be helpful, as the finding of

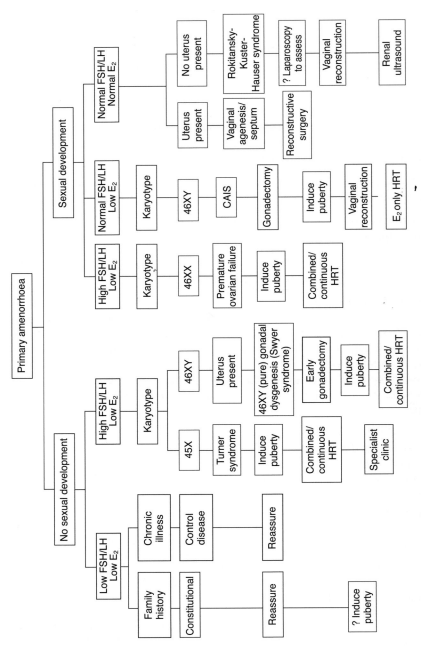

Figure 6.1 Investigation of primary amenorrhoea

follicles in the ovaries is reassuring and confirms the presence of gonadotrophin activity.

No treatment is required for these girls other than reassurance. This is often sufficient, particularly if the mother also had the problem as a teenager. These girls should be followed up, however, to ensure that puberty does occur and that the girl does not wish puberty to be induced.

While the condition is a benign one, it should be remembered that it is often extremely embarrassing for a girl to be significantly less developed than her peers and may result in bullying at school. For these reasons, it may be wise to consider induction of puberty (see later in this chapter).

CHRONIC SYSTEMIC DISEASE

Chronic illness of any type may cause delay in pubertal development. Endocrine disorders, such as type 1 (insulin-dependent) diabetes mellitus or hypothyroidism, are particularly common causes. Other systemic diseases, such as chronic renal failure, congenital cardiac disorders or respiratory conditions such as cystic fibrosis, may also be responsible. In some girls, the systemic disorder may not be recognised. For example, in girls with coeliac disease or gluten enteropathy, failure of pubertal development may be the presenting symptom. Chronic infections such as tuberculosis may also be a cause and should be particularly considered in girls from communities where the disease is prevalent. No specific treatment is required for these girls. Control of the disease is usually all that is required.

Although not strictly classifiable as a 'chronic systemic disease', girls who are emotionally deprived or who have suffered chronic physical or sexual abuse often have delayed development.

ABSENCE OF OVARIAN FUNCTION

Absence of ovarian function may be due to premature ovarian failure or abnormal development of the gonads. Occasionally, girls with PCOS may present with primary amenorrhoea but this will be considered under its more common presentation of secondary amenorrhoea.

Absence of ovarian function is a devastating diagnosis to have to give to a teenager. The main concern expressed by these girls is not so much the fear of disease but the desolation associated with the loss of her fertility. This affects all areas of her life, in particular her relationships at this vulnerable stage.

PREMATURE OVARIAN FAILURE

Ovarian failure may present as primary or secondary amenorrhoea, depending on the stage of development at which the failure occurred. Few studies are available giving statistics for the adolescent age group but premature ovarian failure occurs in 0.1% of women under the age of 30 years.[1] In most cases the cause is not known. In those situations where the cause is known, probably the most common in this age group – and becoming increasingly common – is damage caused by radiotherapy or chemotherapy.

The damage caused by chemotherapy depends on the agent or agents used, the dosage given and the age of the girl at the time of therapy. High doses of alkylating agents cause the most ovarian damage. About 6% of adult female survivors of childhood cancer develop persistent ovarian failure[2] but 96% of women aged between 40 and 49 years develop ovarian failure. In women aged between 30 and 40 years at the time of chemotherapy, the amenorrhoea will be reversed in around 50%.[3] It should be noted, however, that girls who continue to menstruate after chemotherapy are still at risk of premature menopause later in life.

Damage caused by radiotherapy is dose, schedule and age related.[4] A 60% incidence of ovarian failure in women receiving up to 500 rads was reported compared with a 100% incidence of ovarian failure when 800 rads were used.[5] While an overall 6% of women recover normal ovarian function after total body irradiation,[6] 50% of treated prepubertal girls retained adequate ovarian function to enter puberty spontaneously[7] but only 10% treated postpubertally retained ovarian function.[8] The possibility of removal and freezing of ovarian tissue for use in future fertility therapy should be explored, although it should be emphasised that such treatment is still in early development and both the parents and the girl should realise that no guarantee of success can be given.

Uterine damage following pelvic radiotherapy also occurs. Significant reduction in uterine volume has been reported as well as damage to uterine blood flow, although the latter was reversed by giving physiological doses of sex steroids.[9]

Ovarian failure may also be due to genetic or chromosomal causes. Women who are fragile X carriers have a high incidence of ovarian failure,[10] although this does not usually occur as early as adolescence. There is also a higher incidence of ovarian failure in girls who have the karyotype 47XXX. Ovarian failure also occurs in 80% of girls with galactosaemia, direct toxicity of galactose or its metabolites being suggested as the possible mechanism.[11] Deletion of the long arm of the X chromosome is associated with premature ovarian failure. Eight candidate genes for premature ovarian failure have been identified[12] but the full complement of genes on the X chromosome has not yet been identified.

Other causes of ovarian failure include infections such as mumps, particularly when the infection is acquired during fetal life or in the pubertal period and environmental factors, especially smoking, although adolescents have not had a sufficiently long history of smoking for this to be a major factor. Autoimmune disorders have also been implicated, with an increased incidence in disorders such as Addison's disease or the multiple endocrinopathies. Occasionally, ovarian auto-antibodies have been identified in these patients, although the relevance of this is uncertain. One study reported a 39% incidence of autoimmune disorders among women with premature ovarian failure and a normal karyotype[13] and autoimmunity is reported to cause around 40% of cases of premature ovarian failure in women with no detectable chromosomal abnormality.[14]

ABNORMAL GONADAL DEVELOPMENT

Gonadal dysgenesis can be associated with either a 45X or a 46XY karyotype, of which the more common is Turner syndrome. Turner syndrome occurs in one in 2000–3000 live female births and is associated with only one functioning X chromosome. The classical karyotype is 45X but only approximately 50% of these girls have this karyotype on lymphocyte culture, the remainder being mosaic forms such as 45X/46XX or 45X/46XY. Abnormal forms of the X chromosome, such as iso-X or ring X chromosomes, are not uncommon. If chromosome culture is carried out on two tissues the number of girls with the non-mosaic form is reduced to 25%.[15] The importance of using techniques such as fluorescence *in situ*

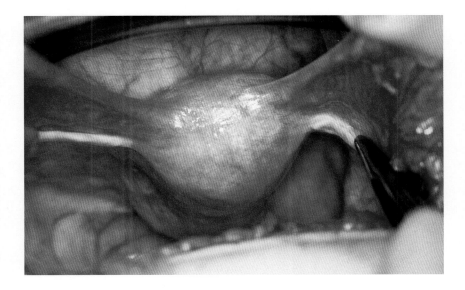

Figure 6.2 Streak ovaries in an adolescent girl with Turner syndrome

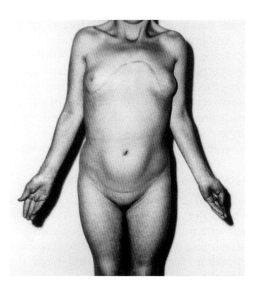

Figure 6.3 Classical appearance of adolescent girl with Turner syndrome (courtesy of Churchill Livingstone)

hybridisation (FISH) in the evaluation of girls with Turner syndrome is emphasised by the finding that one-third of girls with the syndrome tested positive for the *SRY* gene, with the associated potential risks of virilism and malignancy.[16]

Girls with Turner syndrome are believed to have normal numbers of oocytes in the ovary by the fifth month of fetal life. The oocytes undergo accelerated atresia, resulting in few, if any, being present by birth. The ovaries show the classical 'streak' appearance (Figure 6.2). Diagnosis of Turner syndrome is relatively easy in girls with classic signs (Figure 6.3). At birth, diagnosis is usually made by the presence of a web neck, lymphoedema of the hands or feet, cardiac or renal anomalies or coarctation of the aorta. In childhood, the classic symptom is short stature and karyotyping should be part of the standard investigation of such girls. Primary amenorrhoea is the symptom leading to the diagnosis in adolescence.

Owing to the high incidence of mosaic forms of the condition, the phenotype can vary markedly. In the clinic for adult women with Turner syndrome in Liverpool, 54% of women did not have the diagnosis made until the age of 12 years and 21% were not diagnosed until after the age of 16 years (Figure 6.4). A high level of suspicion must be maintained to make the diagnosis in time for the girl to receive optimum therapy, including growth hormone.

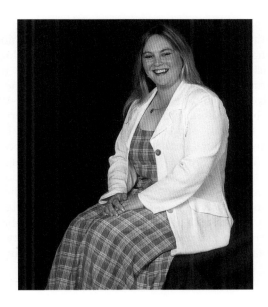

Figure 6.4 Adolescent girl with Turner syndrome showing few of the classical features (with patient's permission) (courtesy of Parthenon Publishing)

Gonadal dysgenesis may also occur in girls with a 46XY karyotype (Swyer syndrome). In these girls, although they are chromosomally male, their testes have been dysgenetic since development and so have produced neither androgens nor müllerian inhibitory factor. This allows the müllerian duct to develop into fallopian tubes, uterus and upper vagina. The presence of female internal genitalia is the differentiating feature between this condition and complete androgen insensitivity syndrome (CAIS) (see below). The uterus may be extremely small due to the lack of estrogen stimulation and it may not be visible on initial ultrasound examination. Repeating the ultrasound examination after induction of puberty will show the uterus clearly.

As the testes in these girls are not only intra-abdominal but dysgenetic, they have a high lifetime risk of becoming malignant (30%)[17] and should be removed as soon as the diagnosis is made.

All women with loss of ovarian function, irrespective of the cause, will have raised gonadotrophin levels and low estradiol levels.

HYPOTHALAMIC PITUITARY DYSFUNCTION

Hypothalamic pituitary dysfunction is a relatively uncommon cause of primary amenorrhoea. Any condition which causes compression of the pituitary or hypothalamus may cause a reduction in secretion of FSH and LH. Such conditions include tumours of the pituitary, craniopharyngioma and hydrocephalus. Other conditions in which the aetiology is less well understood include the Laurence-Moon-Biedl syndrome (an autosomal recessive disorder characterised by obesity, retinitis pigmentosa, mental restriction, polydactyly and hypogonadism) and the Prader-Willi syndrome (characterised by hypotonia, mental restriction, characteristic facies and obesity). The Kallman syndrome, or olfactory–genital dysplasia, is characterised by anosmia, in addition to the lack of secondary sexual development. The anosmia is caused by incomplete agenesis of the olfactory bulbs together with anatomical defects of the hypothalamus. It is thought to be an autosomal dominant condition. In all these conditions, however, it is more likely to be necessary to know that delayed puberty is associated with a previously diagnosed condition rather than looking for such a diagnosis in a girl presenting with delayed puberty. In most girls with hypogonadotrophic hypogonadism, however, the condition is idiopathic.

For all girls with delayed puberty and primary amenorrhoea, in which the cause is not reversible, it will be necessary to induce puberty.

Induction of puberty

The aim of induction of puberty is to mimic the function of the ovary at puberty as much as possible. Treatment should be started about the age of 10 years, although, in girls with Turner syndrome, treatment will probably be delayed to allow maximum response to growth-hormone therapy.

Treatment should begin with small doses of ethinyl estradiol, 1 microgram daily for 6 months, increasing to 2 micrograms, 5 micrograms, 10 micrograms and eventually 20 micrograms, with increments at 6-monthly intervals. Such low doses of ethinyl estradiol are not widely available and arrangements have to be made to obtain supplies of the 2-microgram tablets from specialist units. It is necessary to start at such low doses, as introducing adult levels of estrogen to a prepubertal girl would induce vomiting and dissuade her from continuing the therapy. In addition, it is thought that starting on high levels of estrogen produces abnormal breast development with a firm compact breast with excessive development of the nipple and areola for the underlying tissue, producing an almost oedematous appearance. These changes are irreversible.

On the 20-microgram dose, the girl may experience some breakthrough bleeding and should be made aware of this possibility. When breakthrough bleeding occurs, or when the 20-microgram dose is reached, the girl should be started on a combined estrogen and progestogen preparation.

Practice over Europe varies considerably, both in terms of age of starting therapy and preparations used.[18] There is some evidence to suggest that girls with Turner syndrome who are treated with transdermal estrogen preparations attain a taller final height than those treated with oral preparations – an obvious advantage.[19]

HRT OR THE COMBINED ORAL CONTRACEPTIVE PILL?

The traditional long-term treatment for the older girls has been the combined oral contraceptive pill, which is still the preferred option of most paediatricians. There are, however, grounds for considering one of the wide variety of hormone replacement therapies (HRT) now available as an alternative. Apart from the use of natural, as opposed to synthetic estrogens, the slightly lower dose of estrogen, the lower dose of progestogen and the reduced duration of progestogen therapy with the potential benefits on the lipid profile and cardiovascular system, the most telling reason for choosing an HRT preparation is the longer duration of estrogen therapy needed in such girls.

Using the combined oral contraceptive pill, a girl with absent estrogen production is only receiving estrogen replacement for three weeks out of four, whereas a girl on HRT is receiving continuous estrogen replacement. As these girls frequently have low bone mineral density (BMD),[20] possibly related to a delay in making the diagnosis, it is mandatory that they should receive optimum estrogen replacement. With the advent of the continuous combined HRT preparations, there is the additional option for these girls of 'period-free' estrogen replacement.

The disadvantage is a very real one. Whereas the combined oral contraceptive pill is free of charge, HRT preparations have to be paid for – with a double prescription charge for those who elect to use a cyclical preparation – and while most girls will get their prescriptions free, they will have to pay when they leave full-time education. A further problem is that, while most adolescents would not be embarrassed at their friends finding their prescription for the combined oral contraceptive pill that is not the case for HRT.

Primary amenorrhoea with normal sexual development

The fact that secondary sexual characteristics have developed, shows that the girl has experienced a degree of hormonal stimulation and these abnormalities are normally the result of an anatomical abnormality. Such girls should be investigated by the age of 16 years. It is important, however, to remember that pubertal development is a continuum and that a break in the continuum is arguably more important than empirical figures. A girl of 15 years who began breast development at the age of 10–11 years and still has not attained the menarche needs investigating.

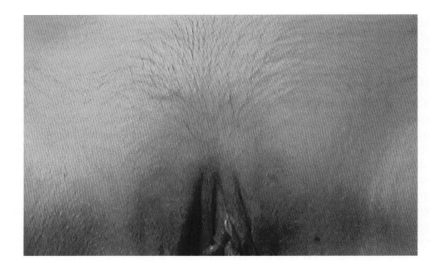

Figure 6.5 Sparse pubic hair in a patient with complete androgen insensitivity syndrome

The main causes are:

- absent uterus or, perhaps more correctly, absent endometrium
- absent or imperforate vagina (more correctly described as cryptomenorrhoea rather than amenorrhoea).

ABSENT UTERUS

Apart from those girls who will have had their uterus removed surgically, absence of the uterus is found in girls whose müllerian duct has failed to develop. This is found in two conditions:

- CAIS (which used to be called testicular feminisation syndrome)
- Rokitansky-Kuster-Hauser syndrome.

COMPLETE ANDROGEN INSENSITIVITY SYNDROME

Girls with CAIS have a normal 46XY karyotype. They have normal female external genitalia, although with sparse pubic hair (Figure 6.5). They have normal testes, no uterus and absent upper vagina – structures that should develop from the müllerian duct. Occasionally, these girls present at birth with bilateral inguinal hernias (Figure 6.6) with the testes palpable. Their phenotype is entirely feminine, classically being slightly taller than average and with good breast development. It is reported that one woman with CAIS is a well-known photographic model.

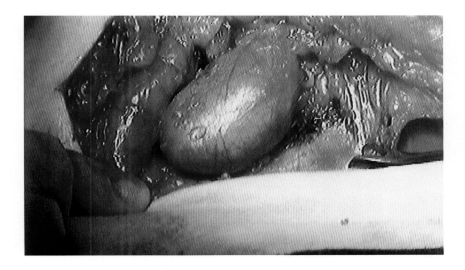

Figure 6.6 Testes at inguinal ring in a patient with complete androgen insensitivity syndrome

The testes in these girls are normal and secrete both müllerian inhibitory factor and androgens *in utero*. The secretion of müllerian inhibitory factor causes regression of the müllerian duct. Close inspection of the introitus reveals only that part of the vagina has developed from the urogenital sinus – usually only a 1–2 cm pouch. Androgen levels are in the high normal male range but the end organ – particularly the skin of the genital area – fails to respond. It is thought that the higher than normal testosterone levels are responsible for the good breast development as peripheral aromatisation to estrogen occurs. The breasts have normal duct and glandular tissue but the areola is often underdeveloped. As well as sparse pubic hair, axillary hair is also sparse. The testes are normal in size, containing Leydig cells, and may be found in the abdomen in the position of normal ovaries, in the inguinal canal or in the labia. Spermatogenesis may or may not be present. As the testes are normal, the risk of malignancy is not as high as with 46XY gonadal dysgenesis, most authorities estimating about 5%.[17]

Genetically, CAIS is caused by point mutations of the androgen receptor gene which maps to the X chromosome at Xg11–12. It is an X-linked recessive condition and a history of an aunt or sister also having the condition is common.

Management of these girls includes gonadectomy and vaginal reconstruction (see below). There is debate about the timing of gonadectomy. As the risk of malignancy is low, some authorities advocate

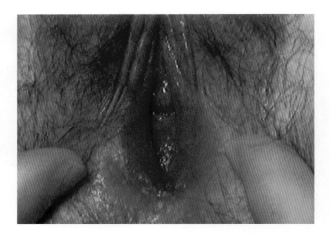

Figure 6.7 Blind-ending vagina in a patient with Rokitansky-Kuster-Hauser syndrome

leaving the testes in place until after puberty to allow breast development. This has the advantage of allowing the girl to participate in decisions about her management. The alternative view is to remove the gonads as soon as possible when the issue will not be such an emotive one for the girl. This would obviously require her to have hormone therapy for induction of puberty (see above). In girls in whom the diagnosis is not made until after puberty, obviously there is no choice. In those in whom the diagnosis is made early because of a family history, the alternatives should be discussed with the girl and her family. Following gonadectomy, long-term estrogen-only replacement therapy is required.

Girls with CAIS and their families require sensitive management, in particular with regard to their sexual status.[21] The practice of gradually responding to the girl's queries (assuming that the diagnosis is known early) is a good one.[22]

Rokitansky-Kuster-Hauser syndrome

Rokitansky-Kuster-Hauser syndrome is the congenital absence of the uterus and upper vagina due to failure of development of the müllerian duct (Figure 6.7) and occurs in one in 4000–5000 births.[23,24] These girls have a normal 46XX karyotype and normal ovaries. Renal, auditory and skeletal abnormalities (particularly hemivertebrae) are common in association with müllerian duct abnormalities.[25]

Occasionally, some rudimentary uterine development, usually without endometrium, will be present and reported on ultrasound scanning, causing problems for the unwary clinician, who will start looking for other causes for the girl's amenorrhoea. If there is no endometrium present, there is no need to remove the rudimentary uterus. These girls require vaginal reconstruction.

Vaginal reconstruction

Vaginal construction may be surgical or nonsurgical. The timing, as for girls requiring gonadectomy, is controversial. Obviously, if a nonsurgical treatment using dilators is to be used, treatment has to be delayed until the girl is old enough to cooperate. Surgical treatment can be performed earlier, the debate once again being related to whether it should be delayed until the girl is old enough to understand the implications of the surgery or whether it should be performed when she is at an age when it will cause her less emotional distress. If dilators are to be used as an adjunct to surgery, surgery should be delayed.

NON-SURGICAL TECHNIQUES

The technique of producing a functional vagina using dilators was first described by Frank in 1938. The potential space between the rectum and the bladder is filled with loose connective tissue and can easily be dilated by the application of a dilator applied to the central dimple. A good vagina can be achieved in this way, particularly if the girl is sexually active, when intercourse can lengthen the vagina. Although a good method, teenagers require a great deal of persuasion to continue as they usually find it rather embarrassing. Having an experienced nurse to help them with the technique and to be readily available for advice is a great advantage.

SURGICAL RECONSTRUCTION

If the use of dilators fails or if there are additional perineal abnormalities that preclude their use, surgical reconstruction will be required. Many methods have been described, including:

- Williams vulvovaginoplasty
- McIndoe procedure, using a split skin graft
- full-thickness skin graft
- vaginal reconstruction using bowel.

Amnion is no longer used because of the risk of HIV infection. All these techniques have their disadvantages, another reason to encourage dilator therapy.

Williams vulvovaginoplasty

The Williams vulvovaginoplasty involves making a 'U' incision from 4 cm on either side the urethra down and round the anus, stitching the skin edges together to form a pouch. While it is the simplest of the surgical procedures, it produces a vagina with a posteriorly directed axis rather than axial and anterior.

McIndoe procedure
In the McIndoe procedure, the potential space above the vaginal dimple is dissected out and a mould covered with split skin from the thigh is inserted. In addition to causing unsightly scarring on the thigh to produce the split skin, the vagina has a tendency to constrict and the girl will have to use dilators throughout her life, during the times she is not sexually active, to prevent the vagina closing. Vaginal dryness has also been reported with this technique.[26]

Full-thickness skin graft
A full-thickness graft does not have the problems of stricture but requires a lengthy hospital stay while the skin of the vulva is expanded using tissue expanders.[27] There is also a risk of hair-bearing skin being introduced to the neovagina.

Vaginal reconstruction using bowel
The technique which probably gives the best result is the fashioning of a vagina by bringing down a loop of bowel on its vascular pedicle through the pouch of Douglas.[28] Sigmoid colon or ileum may be used but the former has the possible disadvantage of causing a heavy mucoid vaginal discharge, which can be offensive.

Cryptomenorrhoea

Girls with an imperforate vagina or, more rarely, vaginal agenesis, but with a functioning endometrium, will usually present with a history of cyclical abdominal pain in association with amenorrhoea, usually about one year after the expected onset of menstruation. The pain is severe and may result in the girl being admitted to a surgical ward with a provisional diagnosis of appendicitis before the correct diagnosis is made. The condition occurs in approximately one in 4000 females.

An imperforate vagina is usually found at the junction of the lower third and upper two-thirds of the vagina at the point where the müllerian duct and urogenital sinus meet. It is caused by the failure of the intervening membrane to break down. The diagnosis may be made in childhood when parting the labia of a newborn girl can show the presence of a hydrocolpos. If the diagnosis is not made at that stage it will not be made until puberty.

In addition to the symptom of cyclical pain, retention of urine may be present, owing to compression of the urethra by the increasing mass. On examination, the girl is found to have a mass arising out of the pelvis. On

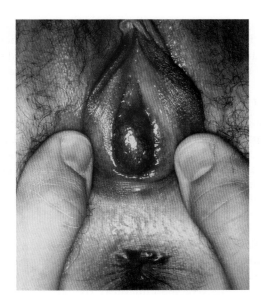

Figure 6.8 Bulging imperforate hymen (courtesy of Churchill Livingstone)

parting the labia, a bulging blue membrane will be seen (Figure 6.8). Treatment is by cruciate incision out to the vagina. It is not necessary to remove redundant tissue of the membrane.

A higher or thicker membrane will not result in the classic appearance of the bulging, blue membrane and may be thicker. Surgical correction will be more difficult and will involve some dissection of the layers to mobilise the epithelium to cover the defect.

Secondary amenorrhoea

Secondary amenorrhoea is defined as the cessation of periods for 6 months or more.

COMMON CAUSES OF SECONDARY AMENORRHOEA

- Pregnancy
- Premature ovarian failure
- Resistant ovary syndrome
- PCOS
- Pituitary disorders
- Hypothalamic disorders.

While pregnancy is obviously the most common cause of secondary amenorrhoea, nothing further will be said about it here. Premature ovarian failure has already been mentioned, the causes and the treatments being the same as for those girls presenting with primary amenorrhoea.

RESISTANT OVARY SYNDROME

Resistant ovary syndrome is a rare condition which presents with the same signs and symptoms as premature ovarian failure and can be difficult to differentiate.[29] In this condition, the ovary contains many primordial follicles which are resistant to the action of high levels of gonadotrophins and do not develop into primary follicles.

Estrogen levels are low, with correspondingly high FSH and LH levels. The differentiating factor between the two conditions is the presence of primordial follicles in resistant ovary syndrome. The use of ovarian biopsy in the differential diagnosis is controversial, however, as the biopsy may not show the follicles and, even if it does, there is no guarantee that the girl will go on to ovulate and menstruate. As, however, there is a remote chance that these girls will spontaneously ovulate, it might be better to consider the combined oral contraceptive pill for hormone replacement if the girl is sexually active.

POLYCYSTIC OVARY SYNDROME

PCOS is an increasingly common but poorly understood cause of secondary amenorrhoea or infrequent periods. The Rotterdam consensus workshop concluded that PCOS is a syndrome of ovarian dysfunction, together with the cardinal features of hyperandrogenism and polycystic ovary (Figure 6.9).[30] The workshop emphasised, however, that PCOS is a syndrome and that a diagnosis should not be based on any single criterion. This is particularly true for ultrasound appearance (Figure 6.10). In addition to secondary amenorrhoea, clinical manifestations of PCOS include hirsutism and obesity.

As the aetiology of PCOS is unknown, treatment is empirical. Weight loss, however, is extremely important, as this reduces the peripheral conversion of estrone and, hence, the circulating levels of LH leading in some cases to a spontaneous return of menstruation. A weight loss of as little as 5% has been associated with improved regularity of menstruation, hirsutism and ovulation and an increased rate of pregnancy.[31] Weight loss has also been shown experimentally to lower insulin resistance and consequently reduce serum insulin concentrations.[32]

For those girls in whom amenorrhoea or highly irregular periods is the main symptom, further treatment is with the combined oral contraceptive pill (COCP). This not only produces a regular withdrawal bleed (which often makes the girl feel happier) but also reduces the long-term risk of

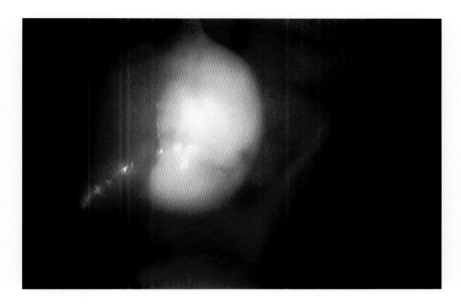

Figure 6.9 Clinical appearances of polycystic ovary

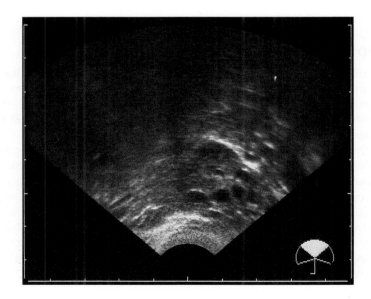

Figure 6.10 Ultrasound appearance of polycystic ovary

endometrial carcinoma. In those girls in whom the hyperandrogenic symptoms (acne, hirsutism) are predominant, the use of the combined oral contraceptive pill containing 2 mg cyproterone acetate is indicated. The girl and her mother should be advised that no improvement in hirsutism will be seen for at least 6 months because of the duration of the average hair cycle and 12–18 months therapy should be allowed for maximum effect.

Increasingly, metformin is being used as a first-line treatment in the management of menstrual symptoms in girls with PCOS,[33] particularly in those with insulin resistance. A Cochrane review comparing the use of metformin with the COCP showed no difference between metformin and COCP in the treatment of hirsutism or acne, but found it to be less effective in improving the menstrual pattern.[34]

It should be remembered that adolescents are extremely conscious of their appearance and that a degree of hirsutism which may not appear severe to the objective clinician can be a major problem for teenagers. While no studies have been done on the psychological consequences of the disorder in this age group, a study in adult women has shown that anxiety and depression are common.[35] This is likely to be more marked in adolescents and this aspect of management should not be overlooked.

PITUITARY DISORDERS

Raised prolactin levels due to prolactinoma are rare in this age group but have been reported.[36] It has, however, also been suggested that cannabis use increases prolactin levels, causing amenorrhoea.[37]

HYPOTHALAMIC DISORDERS

Girls with low body weight as a result of excessive exercise or dieting will have amenorrhoea secondary to hypothalamic dysfunction and low level of gonadotrophin release. Hormone profile shows low levels of FSH, LH and estrogen. When their weight returns to normal, most girls will have resumption of normal menstrual cycles.

In the meantime, however, these girls are difficult to treat. They are at particular risk of osteoporosis because of their low weight, low estrogen and poor diet. Those who are over-exercising are at risk of stress fractures. They usually refuse HRT as they are convinced it will cause them to gain weight. They particularly refuse the cyclical preparations as, especially in the case of girls with anorexia, they may have a desire to remain childlike and so do not wish to have periods. The girl with anorexia also often has a strong desire to be in control and will often exercise that by refusing therapy.

References

1. Coulam CB, Adamson SC, Annegers JF. Incidence of premature ovarian failure. *Obstet Gynecol* 1986;67:604–6.

2. Rutter MM, Rose SR. Long-term sequelae of childhood cancer. *Curr Opin Pediatr* 2007;19:480–7.

3. Hortobagyi GN, Buzdar AU, Marcus CE, Smith TL. Immediate and longterm toxicity of adjuvant chemotherapy regimes containing doxorubicin in trials at MD Anderson Hospital and Tumor Institute. *NCI Monographs* 1986;(1):105–9.

4. Wallace WH, Shalet SM, Crowne EC, Morris-Jones PH, Gattamaneni HR. Ovarian failure following abdominal irradiation in childhood: the radiosensitivity of the human oocyte. *Br J Radiol* 1989;62:995–8.

5. Baker WJ, Morgan RL, Pickham MJ, Smithers DW. Preservation of ovarian function in patients requiring radiotherapy for para-aortic and pelvic Hodgkin's disease. *Lancet* 1972;ii:1307–8.

6. Sanders JE, Buckner CD, Amos D, Levy W, Appelbaum FR, Doney K, *et al.* Ovarian function following marrow transplantation for aplastic anaemia or leukaemia. *J Clin Oncol* 1988;6:813–18.

7. Sarafoglou K, Boulad F, Gillio A, Sklar C. Gonadal function after bone marrow transplantation for acute leukaemia during childhood. *J Pediatr* 1997;130:210–16.

8. Sanders JE, Hawley J, Levy W, Gooley T, Buckner CD, Deeg HJ, *et al.* Pregnancies following high dose cyclophosphamide with or without high-dose busulphan or total body irradiation and bone marrow transplantation. *Blood* 1996;87:3045–52.

9. Bath LE, Critchley HO, Chambers SE, Anderson RA, Kelnar CJ, Wallace WH. Ovarian and uterine characteristics after total body irradiation in childhood and adolescence: response to sex steroid replacement. *Br J Obstet Gynaecol* 1999;106:1265–72.

10. Schwartz, C, Dean J, Howard-Peebles P, Bugge M, Mikkelsen M, Tommerup N, *et al.* Obstetric and gynecological complications in Fragile X carriers. *Am J Med Genet* 1994;51:400–2.

11. Forges T, Monnier-Barbarino P, Leheup B, Jouvet P. Pathophysiology of impaired ovarian function in galactosaemia. *Hum Reprod Update* 2006;12:573–84.

12. Davison RM, Davis CJ, Conway GS. The X chromosome and ovarian failure. *Clinical Endocrinol* 1999;51:673–9.

13. Alper MM, Garner PR. Premature ovarian failure: its relationship to autoimmune disease. *Obstet Gynecol* 1985;66:27–30.

14. Belvisi L, Bombellini F, Sironi L, Doldi N. Organ-specific auto-immunity in patients with premature ovarian failure. *J Endocrinol Invest* 1993;16:889–92.

15. Held KR, Kerber S, Kaminsky E, Singh S, Goetz P, Seemanova E, *et al.* Mosaicism in 45X Turner syndrome: does survival in early pregnancy depend on the presence of two X chromosomes? *Hum Genet* 1992;88:288–94.

16. Kocova M, Siegel SF, Wenger SL, Lee PA, Trucco M. Detection of Y chromosome sequences in Turner's syndrome by southern blot analysis of amplified DNA. *Lancet* 1993;342:140–3.

17. Verp MS, Simpson JL. Abnormal sexual differentiation and neoplasia. *Cancer Genet Cytogenet* 1987;25:191–218.

18. Kiess W, Conway G, Ritxen M, Rosenfield R, Bernasconi S, Juul A, *et al.* Induction of puberty in the hypogonadal girl – practices and attitudes of pediatric endocrinologists in Europe. *Horm Res* 2002;57:66–71.

19. Davenport ML. Evidence for early initiation of growth hormone and transdermal estradiol therapies in girls with Turner syndrome. *Growth Horm IGF Res* 2006;16(Suppl A):S91–7.

20. Garden AS, Diver MJ, Fraser WD. Undiagnosed morbidity in adult women with Turner's syndrome. *Clin Endocrinol (Oxf)* 1996;45:589–93.

21. Personal view. Once a dark secret. *BMJ* 1994;308:542.

22. Goodall J. Helping a child to understand her testicular feminisation. *Lancet* 1991;337:33–5.

23. Griffin JE, Edwards C, Madden JD, Harrod MJ, Wilson, JD. Congenital absence of the vagina. The Mayer-Kuster-Hauser syndrome. *Ann Intern Med* 1976;85:224–36.

24. Lindenman E, Shepard MK, Pescovitch OH. Müllerian agenesis: an update. *Obstet Gynecol* 1997;90:307–11.

25. Strubbe EH, Cremers CW, Willemsen WN, Rolland R, Thijn CJ. The Mayer-Rokitansky-Kuster-Hauser (MRKH) syndrome without and with associated features: two separate entities? *Clin Dysmorphol* 1994;3:192–9.

26. Strickland JL, Cameron WJ, Krantz KE. Longterm satisfaction of adults undergoing McIndoe vaginoplasty as adolescents. *Adolesc Pediatr Gynecol* 1993;6:135–7.

27. Johnson N, Batchelor A, Lilford RJ. Experience with tissue expansion vaginoplasty. *Br J Obstet Gynaecol* 1991;98:564–8.

28. Goligher JC. The use of pedicled transplants of the sigmoid or other parts of the intestinal tract for vaginal construction. *Ann R Coll Surg Engl* 1983;65:53–5.

29. Wentz AC. Resistant ovary syndrome. In: Adashi EY, Rock JA, Rosenwalks Z, editors. *Reproductive Endocrinology, Surgery and Technology.* Volume 2. Philadelphia, PA: Lippincott-Raven; 1995. p. 1385–92.

30. Rotterdam ESHRE/ASRM-Sponsored PCOS Consensus Workshop Group. Revised 2003 consensus on diagnostic criteria and long-term health risks related to polycystic ovary syndrome (PCOS). *Hum Reprod* 2004;19:41–7.

31. White MC, Turner EI. Polycystic ovarian syndrome: 2 Diagnosis and management. *Br J Hosp Med* 1994;51:349–52.

32. Franks S. Polycystic ovarian syndrome: a changing perspective. *Clin Endocrinol* 1989;31:87–120.

33. De Leo V, Musacchio MC, Morgante G, Piomboni P, Petraglia F. Metformin treatment is effective in obese teenage girls with PCOS. *Hum Reprod* 2006;21:2252–6.

34. Costello MF, Shresta B, Eden J, Johnson NP, Sjoblom P. Metformin versus oral contraceptive pill in polycystic ovary syndrome: a Cochrane review. *Hum Reprod* 2007;22:1200–9.

35. Modell E, Goldstein D, Reyes FI. Endocrine and behavioural responses to psychological stress in hyperandrogenic women. *Fertil Steril* 1990;53:454–9.

36. Colao A, Loche S, Cappa M, Di Sarno A, Landi ML, Sarnacchiaro F, *et al.* Prolactinomas in children and adolescents. Clinical presentation and long-term follow-up. *J Clin Endocrinol Metab* 1998;83:2777–80.

37. Teoh SK, Lex BW, Mendelson JH, Mello NK, Cochin J. Hyperprolactinaemia and macrocytosis in women with alcohol and polysubstance abuse. *J Stud Alcohol* 1992;53:176–82.

7 Menstrual problems in adolescents

Problems with heavy or painful menstruation are the most common reasons for seeing a teenager at a gynaecological clinic. It is extremely important when assessing an adolescent with a complaint of abnormal menstruation that a careful history is taken and that some time is spent trying to make an objective assessment of the degree of the problem. It is well appreciated among gynaecologists how difficult it is to do this in adults and it can be more difficult in adolescents, who have fewer criteria against which to measure the degree of their menstrual loss. Failure to do this and to opt for treatment of what is essentially a normal cycle will confirm the girl in her belief that her menstruation is abnormal, with resultant problems in later years. One study, which is rather old now (1966), found a high proportion of girls with adolescent menstrual problems having hysterectomy performed in their early 20s.[1] The mother's fears and expectations also have to be dealt with. The scenario 'I had problems with my periods when I was her age and I ended up having a hysterectomy before I was 30 and my daughter is going the same way' is a well-recognised one which requires sensitive handling. It is important for the girl to understand that she is not necessarily going to have the same problems as her mother.

A normal menstrual cycle is 29 days, with a range of 23–39 days. The average blood loss is 40 ml, with a normal range of 25–70 ml.[2] A blood loss of over 80 ml is abnormal and may result in the teenager becoming anaemic. It is difficult to obtain such objective information, however. Simply asking about cycle length and duration is not helpful. A history that deals with such things as the necessity of getting up at night to change her nightwear or bedding or having to miss school or games because of her periods may give a more accurate picture. One study in a group of adult women complaining of menorrhagia found that 68% had a blood loss of less than 80 ml and in 42% it was less than 50 ml.[3] For some girls, the use of a pictorial chart may be helpful.[4] Keeping a menstrual diary can be extremely useful in the long-term management of these girls.

Heavy and irregular periods

PATHOPHYSIOLOGY

Some understanding of the physiology of menstruation is helpful in the management of teenagers with heavy and/or irregular periods. Whereas in women in their early twenties, 95% of cycles are ovulatory in the first year after menarche, only 15% of girls are ovulating regularly, owing to the failure of the feedback mechanism causing the LH surge.[5] In the early years after menarche, therefore, the endometrium is often under unopposed estrogen stimulation, causing it to become thick and unstable. The endometrium breaks down in an irregular manner, often resulting in extremely heavy menstrual loss. Histology of the endometrium would show a hyperproliferation or simple hyperplasia.

Girls with regular periods are likely to be ovulating. The mechanism for heavy periods in this group is less well understood but is thought to be due to increased endometrial fibrinolysis[6] and an alteration in prostaglandin balance.[7]

It has been noted that the molecular pathways resulting in menorrhagia and dysmenorrhoea have not been well defined and that future research should be done in this area in order to develop better treatments.[8]

MANAGEMENT

Factors in the history should include those mentioned above. There is no role for pelvic or rectal examination in these girls. It is highly unlikely that there will be any uterine pathology and any pelvic abnormality can be identified using ultrasound examination. Pelvic examination is not well received by these girls and insensitive examination may well dissuade them from attending for gynaecological examination, including cervical smears, later in their reproductive life.

Investigations should include haemoglobin estimation. Thyroid function tests may be considered but there is not a great deal of evidence that thyrotoxicosis is a major cause of heavy periods and testing should be limited to those with symptoms of the disease.[9] Ultrasound examination will exclude any ovarian pathology and may provide reassurance that there is nothing seriously wrong. There is no indication for hysteroscopy or dilatation and curettage. Provided that she is not anaemic and that the periods are not causing too much disruption in her life, reassurance for both the girl and her mother may be all that is necessary.

If treatment is required and the girl's periods are regular and heavy, first-line treatment is with the antifibrinolytic, tranexamic acid or a prostaglandin synthetase inhibitor taken during the first 3 days of menstruation.[10] Tranexamic acid 1 g 6-hourly has been shown to reduce menstrual flow by 54% and mefenamic acid 500 mg 8-hourly by 20%.

Tranexamic acid at a dose of 2 g per day has been shown to be effective.[11] Adverse effects of both drugs include nausea, headache and gastrointestinal disturbance.[12] There is no evidence of an increased risk of thrombosis in women taking tranexamic acid.[12] Mefenamic acid has the additional benefit of improving dysmenorrhoea.

Unlike the adult woman, in whom it is unusual to find evidence of hormonal upset,[10] anovulation is commonly a cause of heavy periods in adolescents, particularly in the early years after menarche. This can usually be diagnosed, without the need for hormone assays, by a pattern of extremely irregular periods. Treatment, therefore, with progestogens or with the combined oral contraceptive pill will impose an external cycle, although it must be made clear to the girl that such treatment is not correcting the underlying disorder and that stopping the therapy may result in the recurrence of irregular periods.

The treatment of choice is probably the combined oral contraceptive pill, as it produces better cycle control. However, this may not be acceptable to the girl or her mother as they may perceive this therapy as only being for contraception.

In the event of the combined oral contraceptive pill not being acceptable, treatment with cyclical progestogens may be used. The main adverse effect of the progestogens is weight gain. In addition, C-19 nortestosterone progestogens are more androgenic (resulting in acne and greasy skin) than the C-21 progesterone derivatives. These adverse effects are extremely important to adolescents, for whom appearance is so important. Treatment should therefore begin with C-21 progesterone derivatives, such as medroxyprogesterone acetate or dydrogesterone. These compounds however, are less potent than the C-19 nortestosterone derivatives such as norethisterone acetate, so it may be necessary to change if no improvement is obtained.

The novel progestogen, drospirenone, is a 17alpha-spirolactone derivative and analogue. It has anti-mineralocorticoid and anti-androgenic properties and is now available in COCP and HRT form.[13] It may be a treatment option with an improved adverse-effect profile if it becomes available in a progesterone only preparation.

Whichever treatment is used, the girl should be told to take it for 6–12 months before stopping to see whether her cycle has settled. It is always wise to warn her that there may not have been an improvement and that a suitable time should be chosen (not as she is about to sit important examinations, for example). If her cycle continues to be heavy and irregular, she should be reassured and told to restart therapy for a further year.

In addition to a reluctance to prescribe the combined oral contraceptive because it is giving the wrong message, concern is also expressed about prescribing it to teenagers because of fears that it will cause premature closure of the epiphyses or because of a risk of development of breast cancer in later life. These fears are largely unfounded. By implication, the girl is already producing estrogen when she is menstruating and so epiphyseal closure has already begun and will not be influenced by oral contraceptive usage. Several studies have been carried out on the risk of breast cancer in adolescents taking oral contraceptives. The risk has been defined by the Collaborative Group on Hormonal Factors in Breast Cancer as being 0.5 excess cancers per 100 000 women when used at ages 16–19 years.[14] In girls with proven menstrual problems, this increase has to be balanced against the loss of schooling, the disruption of her lifestyle and the consequences of anaemia. However, an increased risk of breast cancer has been reported with early COCP use in girls who are *BRCA1* and *2* mutation carriers.[15,16] A strong family history of breast cancer should therefore be a relative contraindication to COCP use at a young age and other treatments used as first line.

INVESTIGATIONS: KEY POINTS

- Pelvic examination is not well received by girls.
- Insensitive examination may dissuade girls from attending for gynaecological examinations, including cervical smears, later in their reproductive life.
- Ultrasound examination will exclude any ovarian pathology and may provide reassurance that there is nothing seriously wrong.
- There is no indication for hysteroscopy or dilatation and curettage.

Special situations

ACUTE, HEAVY VAGINAL BLEED

This situation is rare and requires urgent management. Hospital admission is required and a blood transfusion may need to be given, particularly if the haemoglobin is 7 g/dl or less. In addition, hormonal therapy is required. The first line of treatment should be high-dose progestogens. Medroxy-progesterone acetate 10–20 mg 4-hourly should be given for 24 hours. One study using this regimen followed by medroxyprogesterone 20 mg daily for 10 days reduced blood loss in all girls in the study.[17] Intravenous tranexamic acid 1g 6-hourly may also be used. If there is no improvement, or indeed if the bleeding worsens, it may be that the endometrium is so denuded that the arterioles are exposed. In this situation, high-dose estrogen to encourage endometrial proliferation may be given. Regimens reported include conjugated estrogen 0.625–1.25 mg orally every 4–6 hours or 15–25 mg intravenously at 6–12 hourly intervals.[18]

THE GIRL WHO DOES NOT RESPOND TO TREATMENT

Failure to respond to treatment is unusual and should prompt investigation for an underlying cause. An acute bleed at menarche is particularly significant.[19] Leukaemias and blood dyscrasias should have been identified on the initial investigation of full blood count. The role of coagulation disorders is uncertain. One widely reported study of acute adolescent menorrhagia found that 19% of those studied had a coagulation problem, commonly thrombocytopenia or von Willebrand's disease.[20] One study reported 28% (7 of 25) had a clotting disorder.[21] Another study, however, found a much lower rate, with only two girls in the 61 studied having such a disorder.[22]

Tumours of the vagina, cervix and uterus are extremely rare in this age group but estrogen-secreting ovarian tumours have been reported. Ultrasound examination, if not performed at the initial evaluation, should be carried out in all who fail to respond to treatment. Successful treatment with uterine artery embolisation[19] and with recombinant factor VIIa[23] has been reported in severe cases. There may be a role for treatment with GnRH analogues but no cases have been reported in the literature.

THE GIRL WITH LEARNING DIFFICULTIES

Girls with severe learning difficulties present additional problems following the menarche. They may be unable to cope with sanitary protection, resulting in severe soiling. They may also have marked premenstrual mood changes that make controlling their behaviour at such times difficult. In addition, many of these girls are epileptic and have worsening fits premenstrually. There is also a need to watch for drug interactions with anti-epileptic medication (often enzyme inducers) and it may be necessary to consider using high-dose (50 micrograms) ethinyl estradiol preparations. In these circumstances, the aim is usually to produce amenorrhoea. This may be done by administering a continuous combined oral contraceptive pill. Continuous usage will produce amenorrhoea and, once the girl is stable on the therapy, will not interfere with anti-epileptic medication. However, it is usual to have a degree of breakthrough bleeding which should be drawn to the attention of the girl's carers.

Parenteral medroxyprogesterone acetate may be administered. Amenorrhoea may not be achieved immediately but will almost certainly be achieved within 1 year of commencing therapy. Interference with other medication is rare and the potential difficulty of getting the girl to swallow tablets is avoided.

Hormonal implants may be considered if the girl will comply with insertion. These result in amenorrhoea in 41% of users and infrequent bleeding in 24% after 2 years.[24] They have the benefit of having less risk of osteoporosis in long-term use compared with parenteral medroxyprogesterone acetate. This is especially important in girls with mobility problems.

The use of the levonorgestrel-releasing intrauterine system (Mirena®, Schering Health) has been shown to be highly effective in reducing heavy menstrual loss.[25] While this is an effective method, it almost certainly will not possible to insert the device in these girls without a general anaesthetic. As these girls are often small for their age, it might be wise to consider ultrasound measurement of the uterine cavity to ensure that it is long enough to allow the device to be inserted.

DYSMENORRHOEA

Dysmenorrhoea is a common symptom in this age group. In one US study, 59.7% of 2699 adolescents reported some degree of menstrual pain, in 14% of them sufficiently severe as to cause frequent school absenteeism.[26] Dysmenorrhoea is commonly associated with ovulatory cycles, so the usual history obtained is that the dysmenorrhoea began approximately 1 year after menarche. Dysmenorrhoea is caused by increased levels of prostaglandins released by the menstrual endometrium, resulting in increased uterine tone and high amplitude contractions. The pain normally starts either just premenstrually or within the first few hours of the onset of menstruation. It lasts approximately 24–48 hours. It is frequently accompanied by nausea, vomiting, diarrhoea, backache and pain in the thighs. Risk factors identified for the occurrence or severity of dysmenorrhoea in one study included early age of menarche, long menstrual periods, smoking, alcohol and weight over the 90th centile. The authors concluded that the first line of management should be the recommendation to lead a healthier lifestyle.[27]

If medication is required, the first line of treatment is the prostaglandin synthetase inhibitors, particularly mefenamic acid 500 mg three times daily during the first 2–3 days of menstruation. Girls who cannot take antiprostaglandins because of the gastrointestinal effects of the dysmenorrhoea may respond to rectal indomethacin or diclofenac but this is not a favourite route of drug administration among teenagers.

If the dysmenorrhoea is accompanied by heavy periods there may, in addition, be a degree of 'clot colic'. Additional treatment with tranexamic acid as described above may be helpful in these circumstances.

In the event of failure to respond to antiprostaglandin agents or contraindications such as respiratory effects, the combined oral contraceptive pill should be the next line of treatment.

THE GIRL WHO DOES NOT RESPOND TO TREATMENT

Failure to respond to the combined oral contraceptive pill should lead to investigation for underlying causes. Laparoscopy should be considered to

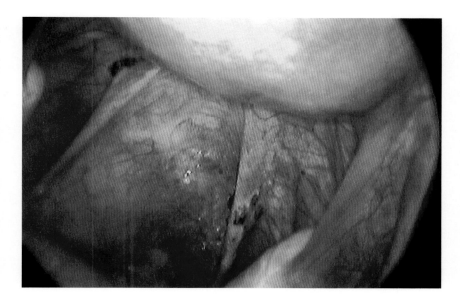

Figure 7.1 Endometriosis involving pouch of Douglas and both uterosacral ligaments in a 17-year-old girl

rule out pelvic pathology such as endometriosis. One study of 140 girls with chronic pelvic pain found endometriosis in 47%, adhesions in 13% and pelvic inflammatory disease in 7%.[28] Another found no abnormality in 40% and endometriosis in 38%.[29] In our own experience, performing laparoscopy on adolescents with dysmenorrhoea which has failed to respond to the combined oral contraceptive pill revealed endometriosis in 50% (Figure 7.1). Of course, with all such diagnoses, it is important to remember that finding such pathology does not necessarily mean that it is the cause of the pain. Also of note is the frequent presence of atypical lesions of endometriosis in adolescents, particularly clear vesicles. These may be early lesions which progress to the usual brown coloured patches but can be missed if not actively sought.[30]

Treatment of endometriosis in adolescents is similar to that in the adult. Destruction or resection of the endometrial deposits at the time of laparoscopy using endocoagulation or peritoneal stripping is possible. Minimal disease, which is amenable to laparoscopic treatment, is most commonly found in adolescents.[30] A Mirena® intrauterine system may be inserted at time of laparoscopy. This has been shown to be effective in the relief of symptoms. As always, screening for pelvic infections, particularly chlamydia, must be performed before instrumentation of the uterus.

Medical treatment includes progestogens, COCP and GnRH analogues.

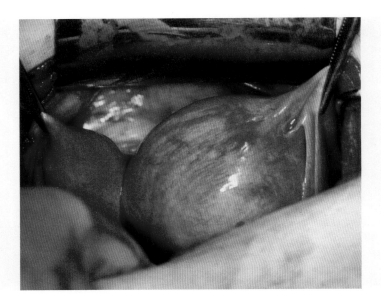

Figure 7.2 Double uterus with distended blind right horn

Use of GnRH analogues is contentious in girls who may not yet have completed their pubertal development. The loss of bone mass, while worrying, has been shown to be reversible.[31] GnRH analogues are well tolerated by adolescents in whom the main complaints are hot flushes, headaches and difficulty sleeping.[32] Alternatively, the use of 'add-back' estrogen/progestogen therapy with GnRH will avoid menopausal symptoms and prevent bone loss although this has not been specifically studied in adolescents.[33]

There is no available evidence to show which treatments, if any, prevent progression of endometriosis and development of adhesions when used in early-stage disease in adolescents. It is not known which treatments are best to protect future fertility.

The other condition that should be considered in girls who fail to respond to treatment for dysmenorrhoea is cryptomenorrhoea. In most girls with cryptomenorrhoea, amenorrhoea is also present and in such circumstances the diagnosis is relatively easy to make. It is much more difficult in those who have a duplex system and therefore appear to be menstruating normally. Ultrasound examination in these girls will usually be reported as showing an 'ovarian cyst' alongside the uterus, which is of course the blind horn of the uterus containing menstrual blood (Figure 7.2). Treatment is by laparotomy to remove the blind horn. A close inspection should be made at the time of laparotomy to ensure that endometriosis is not present. Cryptomenorrhoea is associated with a high incidence of endometriosis. Laparoscopic removal of the blind horn following evaluation by magnetic resonance scan has been shown to be a safe technique in a study of 15 girls.[34]

Ultrasound of the renal tract should also be performed, as it has been reported that malformations of the renal tract are found in up to 47% of women with rudimentary horns.[35]

References

1. Southam AL, Richart RM. The prognosis for adolescents with menstrual problems. *Am J Obstet Gynecol* 1966;94:637–42.

2. Bayer SR, DeCherney AH. Clinical manifestations and treatment of dysfunctional uterine bleeding. *JAMA* 1993;269:1823–8.

3. Cameron IT. Dysfunctional uterine bleeding. *Ballière's Clin Obstet Gynaecol* 1989;3:315–27.

4. Higham JM, O'Brien PMS, Shaw RW. Assessment of menstrual blood loss using a pictorial chart. *Br J Obstet Gynaecol* 1990;97:734–9.

5. Apter D, Vihko R. Hormonal patterns of adolescent cycles. *J Clin Endocrinol Metab* 1978;47:944–54.

6. Dockery CJ, Sheppard B, Daly L, Bonnar J. The fibrinolytic enzyme system in normal menstruation and excessive uterine bleeding and the effect of tranexamic acid. *Eur J Obstet Gynecol Reprod Biol* 1987;24:309–18.

7. Smith SK, Abel MH, Kelly RW, Baird DT. Prostaglandin synthesis in the endometrium of women with ovular dysfunctional bleeding. *Br J Obstet Gynaecol* 1981;88:434–42.

8. Jabbour HN, Kelly RW, Fraser HM, Critchley HO. Endocrine regulation of menstruation. *Endocr Rev* 2006;27: 17–46.

9. Krassas GE, Pontikides N, Kaltsas T, Papadopoulou P, Batrinos M. Menstrual disturbances in thyrotoxicosis. *Clin Endocrinol (Oxf)* 1994;40:641–4.

10. Bonnar J, Sheppard BL. Treatment of menorrhagia during menstruation: randomised controlled trial of ethamsylate, mefenamic acid and tranexamic acid. *BMJ* 1996;313:579–82.

11. Kriplani A, Kulshrestha V, Agarwal N, Diwakar S. Role of tranexamic acid in management of dysfunctional uterine bleeding in comparison with medroxyprogesterone acetate. *J Obstet Gynaecol* 2006;26:673–8.

12. Rybo G. Tranexamic acid therapy is effective treatment in heavy menstrual bleeding. *Clinical Update on Safety Therapeutic Advances* 1991;4:1–8.

13. Fenton C, Wellington K, Moen MD, Robinson DM. Drospirenone/ethinyl-estradiol 3mg/20mcg(24/4 day regimen): a review of its use in contraception, premenstrual dysphoric disorder and moderate acne vulgaris. *Drugs* 2007;67:1749–65.

14. Collaborative Group on Hormonal Factors in Breast Cancer. Breast cancer and hormonal contraceptives: collaborative re-analysis of individual data on 53 297 women with breast cancer and 100 239 women without breast cancer from 54 epidemiological studies. *Lancet* 1996;347:1713–27.

15. Narod SA, Dubé MP, Klijn J, Lubinski J, Lynch HT, Ghadirian P, *et al.* Oral contraceptives and the risk of breast cancer in BRCA1 and BRCA2 mutation carriers. *J Natl Cancer Inst* 2002;94(23):1773–9.

16. Jernstrom H, Loman N, Johannsson OT, Borg A, Olsson H. Impact of teenage oral contraception in a population based series of early onset breast cancer cases who have undergone BRCA mutation testing. *Eur J Cancer* 2005;41(15):2312–20.

17. Aksu F, Madazli R, Budak E, Cepni I, Benian A. High dose medroxyprogesterone acetate in the treatment of dysfunctional uterine bleeding in 24 adolescents. *Aust N Z J Obstet Gynaecol* 1997;37:228–31.

18. Edmunds DK. Dysfunctional uterine bleeding in adolescence. *Ballière's Clin Obstet Gynaecol* 1999;13:239–49.

19. Bowkley CW, Dubel GJ, Haas RA, Soares GM, Ahn SH. Uterine artery embolization for life threatening haemorrhage at menarche: brief report. *J Vasc Interv Radiol* 2007;18:127–31.

20. Classens EA, Cowell CA. Acute adolescent menorrhagia. *Am J Obstet Gynecol* 1982;139:277–80.

21. Oral E, Cagdas A, Gezer A, Kaleli S, Aydin Y, Ocer F. Haematological abnormalities in adolescent menorrhagia. *Arch Gynaecol Obstet* 2002;266: 72–4.

22. Falcone T, Desjardins C, Bourque J, Granger L, Hemmings R, Quiros E. Dysfunctional uterine bleeding in adolescents. *J Reprod Med* 1994;39:761–4.

23. Giovannini L, Appert A, Monpoux F, Fischer F, Boutte P, Sirvent N. Successful use of recombinant factor VIIa for management of severe menorrhagia in an adolescent with an acquired inhibitor of human thrombin. *Acta Paediatr* 2004;93:841–3.

24. Gezginc K, Balci O, Kartayli R, Colakoghi MC. Contraceptive efficacy and side effects of implanon. *Eur J Contracept Reprod Health Care* 2007;16:1–4.

25. Barrington JW, Bowen-Simpkins P. The levonorgestrel intrauterine system in the management of menorrhagia. *Br J Obstet Gynaecol* 1997;104:614–16.

26. Klein JR, Litt IF. Epidemiology of adolescent dysmenorrhoea. *Pediatrics* 1981;68:661–4.

27. Harlow SD, Park M. A longitudinal study of risk factors for the occurrence, duration and severity of menstrual cramps in a cohort of college women. *Br J Obstet Gynaecol* 1996;103:1134–42.

28. Goldstein DP, deCholnoky C, Emans SJ, Leventhal JM. Laparoscopy in the diagnosis and management of pelvic pain in adolescents. *J Reprod Med* 1980;24:251–56.

29. Vercellini P, Fedele L, Arcaini L, Bianchi S, Rognoni MT, Candiani GB. Laparoscopy in the diagnosis of pelvic pain in adolescent women. *J Reprod Med* 1989;34:156–60.

30. Wood PL. Pelvic pain, ovarian cysts and endometriosis in adolescent girls. In: Balen A, editor. *Paediatric and Adolescent Gynaecology.* Cambridge: Cambridge University Press; 2004. p. 359–72.

31. Fogelman I. Gonadotropin releasing hormone agonists and the skeleton. *Fertil Steril* 1992;57:715–24.

32. Bandera C, Brown LR, Laufer MR. Adolescents and endometriosis. *Clinical Consultations in Obstetrics and Gynecology* 1995;7:200–8.

33. Surrey ES. Steroidal and nonsteroidal 'add-back' therapy: extending safety and efficacy of gonadotropin-releasing hormone agonists in the gynecologic patient. *Fertil Steril* 1995;4:673–85.

34. Strawbridge LC, Crouch NS, Cutner AS, Creighton SM. Obstructive mullerian anomalies and modern laparoscopic management. *J Paediatr Adolesc Gynaecol* 2007;20:195–200.

35. Fore SR, Hammond CB, Parker TR, Anderson EE. Urologic and genital anomalies in patients with congenital absence of the vagina. *Obstet Gynecol* 1975;46:410–16.

8   Contraception

With changes in lifestyle and improvements in the standard of living, young people are reaching physical maturity much earlier than in previous generations. As a result of this, adolescents are reaching sexual maturity earlier. Emotional and psychological maturity tends to lag behind, although this is not recognised by the teenager who strives for more independence from the family unit. The rate of teenage sexual activity has increased steadily and consistently over the second half of the 20th century.[1] Young people now start sexual activity at an earlier age and have more sexual partners in their life. Premarital sex no longer carries a stigma and a culture of serial monogamy is now considered by many to be the norm.

Unfortunately, the use of contraception lags behind the increase in sexual activity, with the UK having the highest teenage conception rate in Europe. This prompted the implementation of a Teenage Pregnancy Strategy by the UK Government, combining provision of family planning services with education. This has contributed a steady decline in teenage pregnancy rates from 46.6/1000 in 1998 to 41.3/1000 in 2005.

Sex education

As part of the Teenage Pregnancy Strategy, local authorities were told to prioritise sex and relationship education in schools and charged with developing a comprehensive programme of sex and relationship education in all schools.

Sex education is not based entirely around anatomy and the act of sexual intercourse. The Sex Education Forum recommended that sex education should:[2]

- be an integral part of the learning process, beginning in childhood and continuing into adult life
- be for all children, young people and adults, including those with physical, learning or emotional difficulties
- encourage exploration of values and moral issues, consideration of sexual and personal relationships and the development of communication and decision-making skills
- foster self-esteem, self-awareness, a sense of moral responsibility and the skills to avoid and resist unwanted sexual experience.

Evaluation of the first 4 years of the Teenage Pregnancy Strategy has shown some benefits, with more young people being aware of how to access family planning services and feeling that they are receiving appropriate sexual health education at school. There has, however, not been an increase in the number of people using contraception at time of first sexual intercourse and an increase in the incidence of sexually transmitted infections has been reported.

Social issues

Although premarital sex is now widely accepted, it is still frowned upon by many religions and cultures. Many teenagers still feel uncomfortable about discussing sexual and contraceptive matters with their parents and it is likely that talking to a healthcare professional at a clinic is less intimidating than talking to a parent. To ensure that counselling and advice are easily available, clinics must be sited and timed to allow young people to attend without drawing attention to themselves. Clinics should take place immediately after school or on a Saturday in the shopping centre; informal youth clinics are more acceptable to the young population. To counter the fear of disapproval, these young people should have advice given which is factual and nonjudgemental, giving the young person due credit for seeking advice and ensuring complete confidentiality.

Legality

The legal age of consent in the UK is 16 years. Sexual intercourse with a person below the age of consent is therefore a violation of the law. Prosecutions are rare if both parties are of a similar age. This aspect of legality does not appear to worry teenagers unduly. Their main concern, and a factor in avoiding healthcare professionals, is that they will not be able to obtain contraceptive advice without their parents' knowledge.

A Working Party of the Royal College of Obstetricians and Gynaecologists recommended that 'The health professional has a responsibility to help the young person to understand the implications of sexual activity and the value of confiding in his/her parents. However, it is also important to appreciate that the developing sexuality of young people creates a barrier between them and their parents, which is a part of growing up. A trained responsible outsider may be a more effective source of counselling than the parents'.[3] If a young person aged below the age of 16 years presents for contraception, and if a parent is not present, the suggestion that a parent should be invited to the discussion should be raised. However, if this is not accepted the counselling should continue, respecting the decision of the teenager. At this initial consultation the benefits of delaying sexual activity should be pointed out.

RISKS OF EARLY AGE OF INTERCOURSE

- Increased risk of sexually transmitted disease or pelvic inflammatory disease.
- Increased risk of cervical smear abnormalities.
- Risk of unplanned pregnancy.

If sexual activity is established and the young person wishes to receive contraception, the legal position for the doctor was clearly defined following the case of Gillick vs West Norfolk and Wisbech Health Authority in 1985.[4] The Department of Health provided guidance specifically related to contraceptive provision for those aged less than 16 years[5] and the Law Lords' ruling (Fraser ruling) states that 'a clinician may provide contraceptive advise and treatment to a young person under the age of sixteen without parental consent provided they have confirmed that the young person is competent and that the Fraser criteria are met'.

FRASER CRITERIA

Outline of Fraser criteria which must be met to allow health professionals to provide contraceptive advice or treatment to young people under the age of 16 years without parental consent.
1. The young person understands the advice given.
2. The young person cannot be persuaded to inform her parents or allow the clinician to inform them.
3. It is likely the young person will begin or to continue having sexual intercourse with or without contraceptive treatment
4. The young person's physical or mental health or both are likely to suffer unless she receives contraceptive advice or treatment.
5. It is in the best interests of the young person for the clinician to provide contraceptive advice or treatment without parental consent.

At all times, the young person must have complete assurance of confidentiality.

Contraceptive counselling

All young people need to be given information on the full range of contraceptives available. It is important to remember that all the stereotypical characteristics of the sullen teenager can be found in the teenage patient. The healthcare professional must be nonjudgemental and be able to deal with this type of behaviour. It is important that explicit instructions are given to the young person, as they will often not take any literature home for fear of being found out.

The risk of sexually transmitted disease must be discussed, as it is unlikely that the present relationship will be the only sexual relationship that person and their partner will ever be involved in.

Routine vaginal examinations or cervical smears should not be a prerequisite for contraceptive advice. These procedures are daunting for young people and are unnecessary at early visits as they may actively discourage young people from seeking advice.

CHOICE

It is important to remember that teenagers are very fertile and thus methods recommended need to be reliable. The Faculty of Sexual and Reproductive Healthcare states that age alone should not limit contraceptive choice. Clinicians should aim to maximise a young person's compliance with family planning advice, this is facilitated by providing a wide and appropriate choice of methods. Their sexual activity tends to be spontaneous rather than premeditated, so methods such as the cap are not as effective as in the older population.

CONDOMS

Many young people use condoms as they are easy to obtain, being on sale in chemists and available in dispensing machines in pubs and clubs. Unfortunately, this ready availability means that the young person receives no counselling or instruction in how to use a condom. With adequate instruction, the added advantage of condoms is the protection they afford against sexually transmitted disease. Even if an alternative form of contraception is chosen by the young person, the use of condoms to protect against sexually transmitted disease should be encouraged.

COMBINED ORAL CONTRACEPTION

The combined oral contraceptive pill is the most popular choice among young people, being used by 20% of women aged 16–19 years.[6] They find it convenient and simple to use. Young people are interested in the additional benefits of light periods and the ability to run two packets together to defer menstruation. Long-term benefits appear to be of little interest to the teenage population; their interests are more immediate. Unfortunately, they are also influenced greatly by short-term adverse effects and may stop using the pill if they experience nausea or breakthrough bleeding. One of the main concerns still expressed by teenagers is the worry of weight gain with the combined oral contraceptive pill. However, a Cochrane review has revealed no causal relationship.[7] It is important to explain adverse effects to the young person and initially encourage frequent visits to the clinic to allay fears and possibly change the brand of pill if it seems necessary. One of the most important factors to get across is the difference between risks in a pill cycle and a normal menstrual cycle, in a group who may have been practising their own form of 'natural' family planning using the beginning or end of a cycle as a 'safe' period. Explanation is required to the effect that lengthening the pill-free period by missing pills at the beginning or end of a packet puts the user at risk of pregnancy and that additional contraception using barrier methods is required if the pill-free interval is lengthened for any reason.

The major drawback of the combined oral contraceptive pill is the lack of protection from sexually transmitted diseases, including human papillomavirus, HIV and bacterial infections. Young people should therefore be encouraged to also use barrier contraception.

EMERGENCY CONTRACEPTION

Emergency contraception is an extremely important area of health education, as less than 50% of young people have obtained any contraceptive advice before first intercourse. Thus, the main reasons young people seek advice from contraceptive clinics are the fear of pregnancy following unprotected sexual intercourse or counselling if they have actually conceived. Information on emergency contraception should be given at every visit, whatever method is being used, as UK teenagers who become pregnant commonly express ignorance about available methods.[8]

The oral hormonal method of choice is levonorgestrel. This should be given as a single 1.5-mg dose as soon as possible after the episode of unprotected sexual intercourse and within 72 hours. Young people need to be informed that an intrauterine contraceptive device can be used postcoitally up to 5 days after intercourse. If the timing of ovulation can be estimated it can be used beyond 5 days after unprotected sexual intercourse, as long as it is not fitted beyond 5 days after ovulation.

Whenever a teenager attends requesting emergency contraception, the opportunity should be taken to discuss long-term contraceptive needs. Emergency contraception is now available from a myriad of sources, family planning clinics, GP's pharmacies. NHS 'walk-in centres', although all do not have the ability to provide long-term contraceptive treatment, advice and information should be given.

PROGESTOGEN-ONLY PILL

There appears to be no benefit from the progestogen-only pill in adolescents. The importance of taking this type of pill at the same time each day, with a window of latitude of only 3 hours and the increased incidence of irregular bleeding often lead to discontinuation of the progestogen-only pill in this group. It should not therefore be considered as a first-line method of treatment and is currently used by approximately 2% of young women.

LONG-TERM CONTRACEPTIVES

The increased risks of pelvic infection, menorrhagia and dysmenorrhoea make the intrauterine contraceptive device unsuitable as a first-line contraceptive choice. However, it should still be considered if the girl requires emergency contraception and the hormonal method is unsuitable.

Depot injections of medroxyprogesterone acetate are often tempting for the young woman. Amenorrhoea and a delayed return to fertility do not appear to be a problem to them and the benefit of not having to keep contraceptive supplies hidden from the family are appreciated. However, in some young people the ability to remember an appointment 12 weeks in advance is debatable. The Faculty of Sexual and Reproductive Healthcare has, however, advised that the use of Depo Provera® should be reviewed after 2 years because of the potential adverse effect on bone mineral density. The newer generation of single-rod progestogen-only contraceptive implants do not demonstrate any adverse effect on bone mineral density. The biggest barrier to their use in young people is the ability of the 'clinician' providing contraceptive advice to insert the implant.

There is a large cohort of young people who are now becoming sexually active who previously would not have survived to reproductive age, such as children with congenital heart defects and renal transplant recipients. These young people tend to be well adjusted to their illness and lead normal lives, which includes the same sexual activity as their peers. The consequences to the long-term health of these young women of an unplanned pregnancy or pelvic infection can, however, be devastating. It is incumbent on those health professionals who see them for long-term follow-up to ensure that they have both adequate advice on the possible effects of pregnancy on their condition and advice on suitable contraceptive methods.

References

1. Wellings K, Kane R. Trends in teenage pregnancy in England and Wales: how can we explain them? *J R Soc Med* 1999;92:277–82.

2. Sex Education Forum *A Framework for School Sex Education*. London: National Children's Bureau; 1992.

3. Royal College of Obstetricians and Gynaecologists. *Report of the RCOG Working Party on Unplanned Pregnancy*. London: RCOG; 1991.

4. Gillick v. Wisbech and West Norfolk AHA, 1985: 3 AII ER402HL.

5. Health Services Management. *Family Planning Services for Young People.* HC(FP)86. London: Department of Health and Social Security; 1986.

6. Dawe F, Meltzer H. *Contraception and Sexual Health 2002.* London; TSO; 2003. p. 1–49.

7. Gallo MF, Lopez LM, Grimes DA, Schulz KF, Helmerhorst FM. Combination contraception: effect on weight. *Cochrane Database Syst Rev* 2006;(1):CD003987.

8. Seamark CJ, Pereira-Gray DJ. Teenagers' use of emergency contraception in general practice. *J R Soc Med* 1997;90,443–4.

9 Female genital mutilation

Female genital mutilation is a complex area that raises issues of competing cultural backgrounds, autonomy, health, education and sexuality. Only the medical aspects of female genital mutilation as they relate to teenagers will be considered in this chapter.

Background

Female genital mutilation is practised in many cultures, most frequently in a belt of 28 African countries, with some occurring in the Middle and Far East. With prevalence rates as high as 98% in some countries (Sudan, Somalia), it is estimated that 200 million women are affected.[1] With an increase in migration, female genital mutilation is now encountered in Europe, USA and Australia. While it is most widely associated with the Muslim culture, there is no reference to the practice of circumcision in the Koran. Incidences of the practice in non-Muslim cultures, such as Ethiopian Jews, have been reported. World Health Organization figures suggest that two million women and children have the operation performed every year.[2]

The age at which female genital mutilation is performed varies from culture to culture. In some areas it is carried out at birth. In some parts of Nigeria, it is the custom for the procedure to be performed during the woman's first pregnancy. Most commonly, however, it is carried out in girls before puberty. Immigration figures show that the number of women from communities that traditionally practice female genital mutilation is rising in the UK.[3] Girls from cultures where it is the practice for mutilation to be performed but who live in the UK probably have the operation performed in the country of their family, as there are no reports in the UK of girls being admitted with immediate complications of the procedure. Cases have, however, been reported in the UK of older women having a refashioning of the original circumcision, in some cases with a fatal outcome.[4] It is quite common for girls from countries where the practice is widespread to have been mutilated; gynaecologists seeing adolescent girls from these cultures should be aware of the possibility and should make sensitive enquiries.

The use of language is important. While many prefer the term 'female

Box 9.1	Types of mutilation
Type 1	Excision of the prepuce with or without excision of part or all of the clitoris.
Type 2	Excision of the clitoris and partial or total excision of the labia minora.
Type 3	Excision of part or all of the external genitalia with stitching/narrowing of the vaginal opening (infibulations; Figure 9.1).
Type 4	Unclassified, which includes pricking, piercing or incising of the clitoris and/or labia for cultural/non-therapeutic reasons; stitching of the clitoris and/or labia; cauterisation by burning of the clitoris or surrounding tissue; scraping of tissue surrounding the vaginal orifice (*angurya* cuts) or cutting the vagina (*gishiri* cuts); introduction of corrosive substances or herbs into the vagina to cause bleeding or narrowing.
Variation	While such a classification appears to be precise, the reality is that, with the operation being performed by lay people under far from ideal conditions, the extent of the cutting varies considerably.

genital mutilation' because they feel it a more accurate description of what has been carried out, many women who have undergone the operation and those from their communities find this term emotive and degrading, preferring the term 'female circumcision'. As with all situations in which we deal with something from a culture different from our own, it is

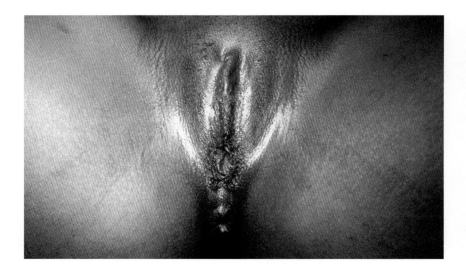

Figure 9.1 Excision of part or all of the external genitalia with stitching/narrowing of the vaginal opening

probably best to ask the girl or her parent how they would prefer the medical team to refer to the procedure.

In the UK, the countries from which it is most common to see girls who have undergone the operation or 'been closed', as it is often expressed, include Somalia, Sudan, Eritrea, Dijbouti, Ethiopia, Sierra Leone and Nigeria.[5] The differing types of mutilation are listed in Box 9.1.

Gynaecological consequences of female genital mutilation

IMMEDIATE COMPLICATIONS

The incidence of immediate complications, such as haemorrhage, pain, urinary retention and damage to surrounding organs, can only be guessed at, as there are no reports in the literature and patients are understandably reluctant to report such problems.

LONG-TERM COMPLICATIONS

Long-term complications are more common in those women who have undergone infibulation. Accurate data are difficult to obtain, as little is written on the subject. One author wrote of Sudanese women that a syndrome of chronic anxiety and depression is common, the latter related to concern over their future fertility, severe dysmenorrhoea and concern about their genitalia.[6]

The most common gynaecological complication is dysmenorrhoea, presumably caused by relative retention of menstrual blood. It should be remembered, however, that dysmenorrhoea is a common symptom in this age group and that mutilation may not be the sole cause. As it is unlikely that permission will be given in this age group for the mutilation to be reversed, treatment should be with nonsteroidal anti-inflammatory drugs. It has been suggested that pelvic inflammatory disease may complicate the retention of menstrual blood but there are no data to substantiate this. Dyspareunia is the most common problem in the older age group and may precipitate a request for the operation to be reversed if this has not been done before marriage.

Many girls experience variable degrees of urinary obstruction, which can lead to poor flow, painful micturition and recurrent urinary tract infections. Other complications include keloid formation in the scar and the development of inclusion dermoid cysts along the scar line. Owing to the prevalence of HIV infection in Africa, there is, of course, an increased risk of the infection among those girls who had the procedure performed there.

The management of pregnancy in women who have undergone either the intermediate type of mutilation or infibulation is an important topic but is outwith the scope of this book.

Legal issues

The Female Genital Mutilation Act was updated in 2003. To date, no criminal prosecutions have been carried out under the Act. Under the terms of the Act, it is an offence for any person to:

- excise, infibulate or otherwise mutilate the whole or any part of the labia majora, labia minora or clitoris of another person; or
- aid, abet, counsel or procure a girl to excise, infibulate or otherwise mutilate the whole or any part of her labia majora, labia minora or clitoris; or
- a person is guilty of an offence if they aid, abet, counsel or procure a person who is not a UK national or permanent UK resident to do a relevant act of female genital mutilation outside the UK.

Some local authorities have incorporated female genital mutilation into child protection procedures and Prohibitive Steps Orders may be invoked which will prevent a child being taken out of the country if it is suspected that the intention may be for genital mutilation to be performed.

The International Federation of Gynecology and Obstetrics published a joint statement with the World Health Organization condemning the practice and calling for it to be abolished.[7]

INFIBULATION

The agreed definition of the word infibulation is that it is 'a stitching together of the labia'. By definition, therefore, when an obstetrician is faced with the repair of the vulva of a woman who has delivered a baby vaginally following a previous infibulation it is illegal then to repair the labia intentionally in such a way that intercourse is difficult or impossible.

Further, although the law states that a surgical operation can be performed on the vulva if the mental health of that person, it states clearly that if a vulval operation is thought necessary for the mental health of that woman, it cannot be performed if only for the purpose of custom or ritual.

Both the Royal College of Obstetricians and Gynaecologists and the Royal College of Midwives interpret the wording of the Prohibition of Female Circumcision Act as including the re-stitching of a previously infibulated woman after delivery. This means that the perineum and vulva can be repaired as medically required but not to such a degree as makes intercourse impossible.

(Royal College of Obstetricians and Gynaecologists press release 1993)

References

1. Dorkenoo E. Combating female genital mutilation: an agenda for the next decade. *World Health Stat Q* 1996:49(2):142–7.

2. World Health Organization. *Female Genital Mutilation: Report of a Technical Working Group*: WHO; Geneva: 1995. p. 9.

3. Foundation for Woman's Health, Research and Development. *Forward Newsletter* November 1998.

4. Khaled K, Vause S. Genital mutilation: a continued abuse. *Br J Obstet Gynaecol* 1996;103:86–7.

5. McCaffrey M. Female genital mutilation: consequences for reproductive and sexual health. *Sex Marital Ther* 1995;10:189.

6. Toubia N. Female circumcision as a public health issue. *N Engl J Med* 1994;331:712–16.

7. International Federation of Gynecology and Obstetrics; World Health Organization. Female circumcision: female genital mutilation. *Int J Gynecol Obstet* 1992;37:149.

10 Gynaecological tumours in childhood and adolescence

Gynaecological tumours are rare in childhood and adolescence. Malignant tumours are fortunately particularly rare. Their rarity, however, may lead to problems, as the diagnosis may not be considered and individual clinicians may have insufficient experience to ensure appropriate treatment.

Childhood cancers differ from those found in adult life in their classification. Those found in the neonatal period are often embryonic tumours, while those in childhood are often sarcomas, as opposed to the carcinomas more frequently found in adult women. This chapter gives an overview of gynaecological tumours in childhood and adolescence only, as their management is extremely specialised and details are not appropriate at this level.

Tumours of the vulva

Tumours of the vulva are particularly rare in this age group. Tumours such as squamous cell carcinoma, malignant melanoma and sarcoma botryoides occur rarely and the only one that even specialists may see is haemangioma.

HAEMANGIOMA

Haemangiomas used to be classified as being either capillary or cavernous but this classification has now been abandoned. They are not usually present at birth but appear within a few weeks, undergoing a phase of rapid growth before undergoing spontaneous involution, although the time period for this is usually rather long.

Haemangiomas are composed, in the early stages, of proliferating masses of endothelial cells with occasional lumina, later, as they resolve, developing into large endothelial lined spaces. Haemangioma of the vulva, as elsewhere on the body, may be superficial or deep. Superficial lesions appear initially as an area of pallor appearing in the first few weeks of life, which develops into a telangiectatic patch, eventually becoming a bright red, well-demarcated, lobulated tumour. The growth of these tumours is rapid over the first 6 months of life, slowing down thereafter, with little growth occurring after 10 months of age. Involution produces greyish coloured areas within the tumour and is usually complete by the age of 9–10 years, although vulval tumours may take longer to disappear than those found elsewhere on the body.

Deeper lesions have a similar growth and involution pattern but appear as soft bluish elevated tumours that are less well demarcated than the superficial type.

Management is largely by reassurance that the tumours will resolve, although active intervention may be required in a few, potentially complicated cases.

Other conditions, such as hymeneal cysts and tags, urethral prolapse, hydroceles and hydrocolpos may all appear as tumours or masses on the vulva or at the introitus. Bartholin's cysts are extremely uncommon in this age group.

Tumours of the vagina

The well-known tumour of the vagina in this age group is now rarely seen: the clear-cell adenocarcinoma related to vaginal adenosis and exposure to diethylstilboestrol (DES) in utero. The association between DES and these conditions was first reported by Herbst and Scully in the early 1970s.[1] This drug, which was never widely used in the UK, had been advocated in the late 1940s for the prevention of miscarriages, preterm labour, pregnancy-induced hypertension and stillbirth.[2] It was estimated that the risk of DES-exposed girls developing clear-cell adenocarcinoma was between 0.14/1000 and 1.4/1000.[3]

Vaginal adenosis is the presence of glandular tissue in or under the vaginal epithelium, which causes a 'heaped up' appearance. The tissue is initially red in colour but undergoes squamous metaplasia, becoming a normal pale pink colour. Dysplastic change may occur within the area of squamous metaplasia. Although historically linked with DES exposure, it may occur without such stimulation. The condition is usually asymptomatic and found by chance on examination. If symptoms do occur, the most common is discharge. Sexually active girls may complain of dyspareunia or, more commonly, postcoital bleeding. Management is usually expectant but treatment by means of excision may be required if the bleeding is profuse.

DES exposure in utero may also cause a variety of structural genital tract abnormalities, including uterine hypoplasia, cervical hoods, pseudopolyps and cockscomb deformity of the cervix.

CLEAR-CELL ADENOCARCINOMA

Clear-cell adenocarcinoma presents in the same way as vaginal adenosis, with discharge and postcoital bleeding, although it may be asymptomatic, particularly in the early stages. Macroscopically, the tumour appears as a firm polypoid lesion, usually anteriorly and in the upper third of the vagina, which may be ulcerated. The tumour spreads locally, to the adjacent vagina and cervix and to the lymph nodes. Microscopically, the tumour consists of clear cells with tubules and cysts lined by the characteristic 'hobnail' cells.

Treatment is by radical surgery with adjunctive radiotherapy, dependent on staging, although wide local excision accompanied by lymphadenectomy and radiotherapy has been reported as a successful combined method of treatment for those girls with tumours less than 2 cm in diameter.[4] The 5-year survival rate is reported as 90% for those with stage I disease but is poor for those with advanced disease.

The number of cases of clear-cell adenocarcinoma of the vagina has declined steadily, particularly in the USA, since DES was banned by the US Food and Drug Administration in 1971.

GARTNER'S DUCT CYSTS

Gartner's duct cysts are embryological cysts deriving from the mesonephric duct. They are quite common and are found in the anterolateral aspect of the vagina, anywhere from the cervix to the introitus. They are usually asymptomatic but may cause dyspareunia. They only require to be removed if they are symptomatic. Treatment is by marsupialisation.

Tumours of the cervix

SARCOMA BOTRYOIDES

The most common tumour of the cervix and vagina in children and adolescents under the age of 16 years is sarcoma botryoides.[5] It occurs most commonly below the age of 2 years, with 90% of the tumours occurring in girls below the age of 5 years. The tumour arises most commonly from the vagina in young girls and from the cervix in older girls and adolescents.

Symptoms are vaginal bleeding and bloody discharge. In young girls the tumour may be seen protruding from the introitus while in older girls an abdominal mass may be present.

The tumour is a highly malignant rhabdomyosarcoma, which originates in the subepithelial layer of the vagina or cervix. The tumour spreads to the posterior vaginal wall, the bladder and the urethra. Later spread is by blood and lymphatics to the lung, liver and bone. Macroscopically, the tumour has a characteristic polypoid appearance, said to resemble a bunch of grapes, and is usually situated on the anterior vaginal wall. The colour may vary from pale pink to dark red. The tumour is subepithelial and has normal epithelium over it, giving it a remarkably benign appearance and so the diagnosis may be missed, even on biopsy, if the deeper epithelial structures are not included in the biopsy.

Microscopically, the tumour consists of poorly differentiated spindle cells, oedematous stroma and large vacuolated, multinucleated, eosinophilic cells known as rhabdomyoblasts. Striated muscle cells may also be present.

Diagnosis is made by examination under anaesthesia, with proctoscopy and cystoscopy included, and biopsy. Examination under anaesthesia should be performed, even in those patients in whom the tumour is seen at the vulva, so that the degree of local spread can be evaluated.

Treatment is with triple chemotherapy (vincristine, actinomycin D and cyclophosphamide) to shrink the tumour mass, with or without radiotherapy, depending upon the response. The residual disease is then removed surgically, by hysterectomy and vaginectomy, with additional chemotherapy for a further 18–24 months. Survival rates following this multimodal regimen are good.

Conservative treatment, particularly for vulval and vaginal sarcoma botryoides, has been reported, allowing the girl to retain her reproductive function.

OTHER MALIGNANT TUMOURS

Other malignant tumours of the cervix in this age group are almost unknown. Benign cervical polyps are also rare.

Tumours of the uterus

Uterine tumours, whether benign or malignant, are extremely rare in childhood and adolescence.

Tumours of the ovary

Ovarian tumours are the most common genital tract tumours in girls and adolescents although they account for no more than 1% of all tumours found in girls under the age of 16 years. The most common ovarian tumour in this age group is ovarian teratoma, which accounts for approximately 30% of the total.

Fetal and neonatal ovarian cysts

Fetal ovarian cysts may be found as an incidental finding on ultrasound examination during pregnancy. They usually develop in response to the high levels of maternal human chorionic gonadotrophin. They require no treatment unless they are of such a size as compromise fetal lung development. In the neonatal period, treatment is similarly expectant.

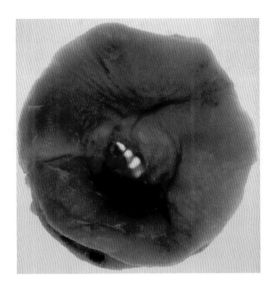

Figure 10.1 Ovarian teratoma with tooth formation (courtesy of Edward Arnold)

Complications have only been reported in cysts over 5 cm in diameter.[6] Treatment of cysts over 5 cm should be by simple aspiration with ultrasound follow-up. Surgery should be reserved for recurrent cysts and those with complications.

Many ovarian cysts in childhood are asymptomatic. Symptoms, when they do occur, include abdominal pain, which may be periumbilical in younger girls, or the presence of an abdominal mass.

FUNCTIONAL OVARIAN CYSTS

Functional ovarian cysts, including follicular cysts and corpus luteum cysts (in girls who are ovulating), should be treated as outlined above.

Benign tumours and neoplasia

TERATOMA

Teratoma is the most common benign ovarian tumour in girls and young women, with the median age of occurrence being 30 years.[7] They are usually less than 10 cm in diameter and appear on ultrasound as partly solid, partly cystic structures. Areas of calcification may also be seen (Figure 10.1).

Teratomas are derived from totipotential primordial germ cells and derivatives of all three germ layers may be found. The most common elements are squamous epithelium, containing sebaceous glands, often also with sweat glands and hair follicles. Cutting into such a tumour releases hair and sebaceous material, giving rise to the common name 'dermoid cyst'; this type accounts for approximately 97% of these tumours.

Treatment is by excision with close inspection of the other ovary as 10–15% of these tumours are bilateral either at the time of presentation or later in life. In view of this, every attempt should be made to preserve ovarian tissue from the affected ovary. The risk of recurrence following conservative surgery is low.

Thyroid tissue is a not unusual component of teratomas, occurring in 5–20% of tumours. Such thyroid tissue may be active and may give rise to symptoms of thyrotoxicosis. Teratomas which are largely or completely composed of thyroid tissue are known as 'struma ovarii'.

MUCINOUS CYSTADENOMA

This is the most common tumour found in adults and may therefore present in older adolescents. They can be extremely large in size, filling the whole abdominal cavity. Ultrasound examination shows a multiloculated cyst. Histologically, the cysts are lined with columnar epithelium. At laparotomy, they are found to contain mucinous material. Great care must be taken when removing these tumours as, if the cysts rupture, with release of the mucinous material, the girl may develop 'pseudomyxoma peritonei', recurrent deposits of mucinous-producing cells in the abdomen which can be difficult to clear, despite repeated surgery, and which may prove fatal.

SEROUS CYSTADENOMA

These tumours are less commonly found in adolescents. They are not as large as their mucinous counterparts, rarely being larger that 15 cm. Ultrasound examination shows a unilocular or occasionally multilocular cyst. Macroscopically, the serous cystadenoma may be lined with papillary excrescences, which may appear on the outer surface of the tumour, giving a falsely malignant appearance to the tumour. Microscopically, the cyst is lined with tall, ciliated columnar epithelium.

Sex cord tumours

GONADOBLASTOMA

This uncommon tumour, which consists of germ-cell and sex-cord stromal elements, is found in adolescents and young women, usually those with a Y chromosome or a portion of a Y chromosome, in their karyotype. The

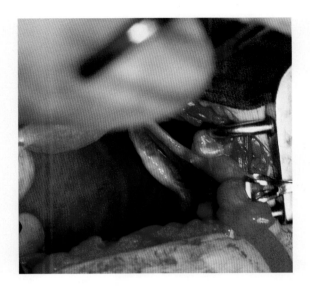

Figure 10.2 Gonadoblastoma in a 15-year-old girl with 46XY gonadal dysgenesis

tumour is benign but as germ cells are a frequent component, a dysgerminoma may develop. Gonadoblastomas are small smooth tumours (Figure 10.2), which histologically show islands of germ cells mixed with smaller sex cord cells. Calcification is a feature. Approximately one-third of these tumours are bilateral, but irrespective of whether they are unilateral or bilateral at laparotomy, both gonads should be removed.

FIBROMA

Fibromas are rare in girls and adolescents. They are small, solid tumours which histologically are composed of bundles of spindle cells.

THECOMA AND GRANULOSA CELL TUMOUR

Thecoma and granulosa cell tumours are rare before puberty. Thecomas are of significance as, although rare, 70% of them will present as precocious puberty.[8] Treatment is by unilateral oophorectomy.

SERTOLI-LEYDIG CELL TUMOURS

Sertoli-Leydig cell tumours are also rare in childhood and adolescence but are significant as they may present with virilisation. As they are of low malignant potential, treatment is by unilateral oophorectomy.

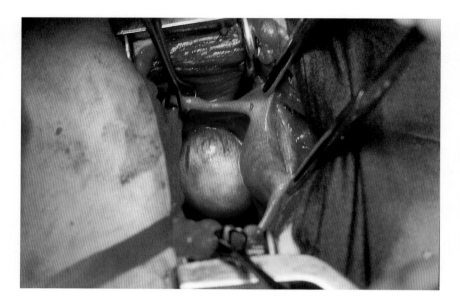

Figure 10.3 Dysgerminoma in the same patient as Figure 10.2

Malignant ovarian tumours

The most common malignant ovarian tumours in this age group are the germ-cell carcinomas, with approximately two-thirds of malignant ovarian tumours in this age group being germ cell in origin. The common ones which occur are dysgerminoma, endodermal sinus tumour, malignant teratoma and, more rarely, embryonal carcinoma, primary ovarian choriocarcinoma and mixed germ cell tumour.

As in the adult group, the main presenting symptoms are pain and the presence of a mass although, in young girls, more non-specific symptoms of urinary frequency, rectal discomfort and abdominal fullness with loss of appetite may be found.

DYSGERMINOMA

Dysgerminoma is the most common malignant ovarian tumour in childhood and young women, with 60% of these tumours being found in the under 20-year age group. The tumour is usually unilateral, with 10–15% of patients having bilateral tumours. Ultrasound examination shows a solid tumour which may be up to 15 cm in size. Macroscopically, the tumour has a white/cream capsule and is round, smooth and lobulated (Figure 10.3). Areas of cystic degeneration, haemorrhage or necrosis are frequently present. Microscopically, dysgerminomas consist of clusters of large neoplastic cells, with irregular nuclei and abundant, pale cytoplasm, arranged in cords or nests with intervening strands of connective tissue. Lymphocytic infiltration of the connective tissue strands, occasionally with eosinophils, is present. Pure dysgerminomas do not produce any tumour markers but coexistent areas of choriocarcinoma, endodermal sinus tumour or malignant teratoma may be present and may produce hCG or alphafetoprotein (AFP).

Treatment is by surgical excision, which in young girls with early disease may be unilateral oophorectomy, unless the girl has a Y chromosome in her karyotype. However, as the tumour in the contralateral ovary may be very small, it may prudent to consider taking a biopsy, taking care not to damage its blood supply. Palpable para-aortic or pelvic lymph nodes should also be removed or biopsied.

Residual disease may be treated by radiotherapy or chemotherapy as the tumour is extremely sensitive to both. Chemotherapy using the platinum group of drugs is increasingly being used as the treatment of choice, so as to maintain residual ovarian function.

Five-year survival rates for pure dysgerminomas are 90–95%. If, however, other tumour elements are present such as endodermal sinus tumour, then the prognosis is influenced by the most malignant component of the tumour.

ENDODERMAL SINUS TUMOUR

Endodermal sinus tumour, which used to be called a yolk-sac tumour, is an extremely aggressive malignant tumour. The tumour is almost exclusively one of adolescents, with a median age of presentation of 19 years.[9] Whereas all malignant ovarian tumours may present with pain, this is a typical presentation of an endodermal sinus tumour because of its rapid growth. Ultrasound examination shows a large solid tumour, usually over 10 cm in size, often with cystic areas due to necrosis. Macroscopically, endodermal sinus tumours appear as grey or yellow encapsulated, smooth but nodular tumours. Degeneration, necrosis and haemorrhage are common. It is not uncommon for them to rupture because of the friable nature of the tumour. Microscopic examination shows a variety of patterns, of which the microcystic is the most common. Schiller-Duval bodies (a central capillary in a mesenchymal core surrounded by cuboidal tumour cells and projecting into the microcysts) are a classical finding. The tumour may secrete AFP, which can then be used as a marker to monitor treatment. hCG levels may also be elevated if other tumour elements are present.

Treatment in this age group is by unilateral oophorectomy with adjuvant chemotherapy using the platinum group of drugs and bleomycin.

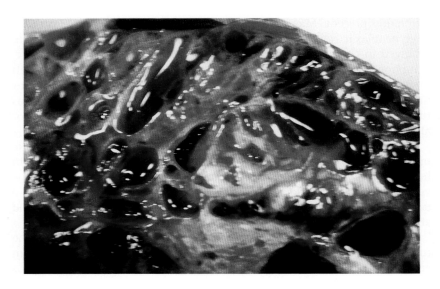

Figure 10.4 Embryonal carcinoma from a 14-year-old girl showing multiple cyst formation

MALIGNANT TERATOMA

The more common form of malignant teratoma in this age group is the immature teratoma, with embryonic forms of all three germ-cell layers being present. Neuroectodermal tissue is the most common component. Approximately 8% of all ovarian tumours in girls under 15 years of age are immature teratomas.[10] Ultrasound appearances are similar to the mature teratoma, with cystic and solid areas being present. Tumour markers are usually negative unless choriocarcinoma is present, when hCG levels will be raised.

Treatment is by surgical removal with sampling of peritoneal implants, which may be of a different histological grading than the original tumour. Adjuvant chemotherapy is used postoperatively. Prognosis is dependent on the size of the tumour, the completeness of resection and the amount of immature tissue present.

Malignant change in one of the elements of a mature teratoma is rare in this age group.

EMBRYONAL CARCINOMA

The median age of presentation of embryonal carcinoma is 14 years.[11] It is rare but aggressive, vying with endodermal sinus tumour for being the most aggressive ovarian tumour of childhood. The tumour is large and solid but cystic areas may be seen on scan due to necrosis and result in the tumour being soft to touch (Figure 10.4). Microscopically, the tumour consists of pleomorphic epithelial like cells with eosinophilic cytoplasm. The tumour may secrete both AFP and hCG. Treatment is by surgical excision with adjuvant chemotherapy using the platinum preparations.

CHORIOCARCINOMA

Choriocarcinoma is an extremely rare tumour with a poor prognosis which secretes hCG. Treatment, as with the other germ cell tumours, is by surgical excision and adjuvant chemotherapy using a platinum combination.

References

1. Herbst AL, Scully RE. Adenocarcinoma of the vagina in adolescence: a report of seven cases including six clear cell carcinomas (so called mesonephromas). *Cancer* 1970;25:745–57.

2. Smith OW. Diethylstilboestrol in the prevention and treatment of complications of pregnancy. *Am J Obstet Gynecol* 1948;56:821–34.

3. Herbst AL. Current status of the DES problem. *Obstet Gynecol Surv* 1979;34:844–50.

4. Senekjian EK, Frey FW, Anderson D, Herbst AL. Local therapy in stage I clear cell adenocarcinoma of the vagina. *Cancer* 60, 1987;1319–24.

5. Copeland LJ, Gershenson DM, Saul PB, Sneige N, Stringer CA, Edwards CL. Sarcoma botryoides of the female genital tract. *Obstet Gynecol* 1985;66:262–6.

6. Widdowson DJ, Pilling DW, Cook RCM. Neonatal ovarian cysts: therapeutic dilemma. *Arch Dis Child* 1988;68:737–42.

7. Surti U, Hoffner L, Chakravariti A, Ferrell RE. Genetics and biology of human ovarian teratoma. I: Cytogenetic analysis and mechanism of origin. *Am J Hum Genet* 1990;47:635–43.

8. Young RH, Dickersin GR, Scully RE. Juvenile granulosa cell tumour of the ovary. A clinic-pathological analysis of 125 cases. *Am J Clin Path* 1984;8:575–96.

9. Gerherson DM, del Junco G, Herson J, Rutledge FN. Endodermal sinus tumour of the ovary: the MD Anderson experience. *Obstet Gynecol* 1983;61:194–202.

10. Neven P, Shepherd JH, Lowe DG. Gynaecological malignancies in childhood.In: Studd JWW, Jardine-Brown C, editors. *Yearbook of the Royal College of Obstetricians and Gynaecologists, Volume 1*. London: RCOG Press; 1993. p. 157–67.

11. Kurman RJ, and Norris HJ, Endodermal sinus tumour of the ovary. *Cancer* 1976;38:2404–19.

Index

Streptococcus pyogenes 20
struma ovarii 104
swabs
  child sexual abuse 46–7
  recurrent bacterial vulvovaginitis 20,
    22
Swyer syndrome 57

Tanner stages of pubertal development
    3, 4–5
Teenage Pregnancy Strategy 85–6
teratoma, ovarian 102, 103–4
  immature 108
  malignant 108
testes
  complete androgen insensitivity
    syndrome 61–2
  development 7–8
  dysgenetic 57
  undermasculinised males 13–14
testicular feminisation syndrome see
    complete androgen insensitivity
    syndrome
testis-determining factor (TDF) 7
testosterone 7–8, 13
thecoma 105
thelarche, premature 33, 34
threadworms 23
thyrotoxicosis 74, 104
tranexamic acid 74–5, 76, 78
trauma, genital tract 28
tuberculosis 53
tumours, gynaecological 99–109
Turner syndrome 55–6, 57
  treatment 58, 59

undermasculinised males 11–12, 13–14
urethral prolapse 100
urinary complications, female genital
    mutilation 95
urinary retention 64
urogenital sinus 10
uterus
  absent 60–4
  double, dysmenorrhoea 80–1
  growth and development 5
  radiotherapy-induced damage 54
  tumours 102

vagina
  adenosis 100
  agenesis 64
  dilators 63
  epithelial appearances 4, 18
  flora, prepubertal child 20
  foreign bodies 27–8
  imperforate 64–5
  reconstruction 63–4
  tumours 100–1
vaginal bleeding
  acute heavy 76–7
  premature menarche 34
  prepubertal child 2, 26–8
  tumours causing 101
vaginal discharge 17–22
vaginal examination 88
Vaniqa® cream 38
virilism 36, 39
vulva
  dermatological conditions 23–4
  irritation without discharge 22–5
  tumours 99–100
vulvitis, non-specific 25
vulvovaginitis 17
  recurrent bacterial 17–22

weight
  loss, polycystic ovary syndrome 66
  low, amenorrhoea 68
  at menarche 1–2
Williams vulvovaginoplasty 63–4
wolffian ducts 8

X chromosome
  abnormal forms 55
  deletion of long arm 54
XXX karyotype 54
XY females 57, 104–5, 107

yolk-sac tumour 107